Nursing Ethics

A Virtue-Based Approach

Alan E. Armstrong
Senior Lecturer, University of Central Lancashire, UK

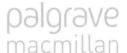

First published in hardback 2007
This paperback edition published 2010 by
PALGRAVE MACMILLAN

Palgrave Macmillan in the UK is an imprint of Macmillan Publishers Limited, registered in England, company number 785998, of Houndmills, Basingstoke, Hampshire RG21 6XS.

Palgrave Macmillan in the US is a division of St Martin's Press LLC, 175 Fifth Avenue, New York, NY 10010.

Palgrave Macmillan is the global academic imprint of the above companies and has companies and representatives throughout the world.

Palgrave® and Macmillan® are registered trademarks in the United States, the United Kingdom, Europe and other countries.

ISBN 978-0-230-50688-6   hardback
ISBN 978-0-230-24419-1   paperback

This book is printed on paper suitable for recycling and made from fully managed and sustained forest sources. Logging, pulping and manufacturing processes are expected to conform to the environmental regulations of the country of origin.

A catalogue record for this book is available from the British Library.

Library of Congress Cataloging-in-Publication Data
Armstrong, Alan E., 1967-
    Nursing ethics : a virtue-based approach / Alan E. Armstrong.
        p. cm.
    Includes bibliographical references and index
        ISBN-13: 978-0-230-50688-6 (cloth) 978-0-230-24419-1 (pbk)
        1. Nursing ethics.   I. Title.
RT85A76 2007
174.2—dc22   2006052517

10   9   8   7   6   5   4   3   2   1
19   18   17   16   15   14   13   12   11   10

Printed and bound in Great Britain by
CPI Antony Rowe, Chippenham and Eastbourne

Contents

Preface and Acknowledgements

This book is based on my PhD thesis, which was awarded to me by the University of Newcastle upon Tyne, UK, in 2004. My professional background as a qualified nurse motivated a deep interest in ethics, which I later studied at BA and MA level; both courses were taught using a philosophical approach to ethics. Therefore, I decided not to base my PhD thesis on an empirical research study. Instead, I attempted to propose a philosophical argument about the value of the moral virtues and apply this to contemporary nursing practice. That, in a nutshell, is the topic of this book.

There is one stylistic issue worth mentioning: I have tried to be consistent with nomenclature; I use words such as 'people' and 'persons' in the Chapters dealing with general ethics and tend to use 'patient(s)' in the Chapters that deal with nursing ethics and nursing practice.

There are many people that I would like to thank because without their help, this book would never have been completed. In no particular order, I thank Dr Shaun Parsons for his help in supervising my PhD thesis. The majority of this book was written while on sabbatical from my post as a senior lecturer in nursing at the University of Central Lancashire, Preston, UK. I would like to thank my divisional leader, Mrs Sheelagh Greenham, and head of department, Dr Bernard Gibbon, for their help and support over the past few years and, in particular, their help in applying for the sabbatical. I would like to thank Daniel Bunyard at Palgrave Macmillan for his help throughout the book-writing process. I owe a great deal of gratitude to my immediate family, my parents, Kenneth and Mary, my sister, Dawn and my brother-in-law, Steven. I have benefited greatly because of their love and friendship, not to mention financial help a few years ago! I would like to thank my stepdaughter, Stephanie; it is fortunate that we get on very well together, we have shared lots of laughs and she has understood how I have needed to dominate the PC! Last but certainly not least, it is difficult to express in words my gratitude and love for my wife, Carol. Since the day we met (16 April 1999), we have always enjoyed ourselves, she has helped me to understand myself more and given me more love and support than I probably have deserved. I dedicate this book to Carol, my beautiful wife.

An overview of this book was published by Blackwell in 2006: Armstrong, A. E. Towards a strong virtue ethics for nursing practice, *Nursing Philosophy*, 7(3), 110–24.

1
Introduction

Broad aim of the book

In this book, I critique examples of act-centred obligation-based moral theories and I conclude that traditional versions of these theories are incomplete and inadequate for use as a nursing ethics. Instead, I argue that a virtue-based approach to moral decision-making provides a more defensible and plausible nursing ethics.

Plan of the book

This book consists of 11 chapters, which I shall now outline.

Chapter 2 – Illness, Narratives and the Value of the Nurse–Patient Relationship

I begin by examining several important themes in contemporary nursing practice. These themes are illness and narratives, hospitalization and patients' emotions, the history of the nurse–patient relationship, contemporary views of empowerment and the nurse–patient relationship, the 'therapeutic' or 'helping' nurse–patient relationship, the role of the nurse and possible definitions of a 'good' nurse.

Chapter 3 – The Virtues in General Ethics

One of the conclusions drawn in Chapter 2 relates to the importance of morally good character traits, which are more accurately called the virtues. Hence in this chapter, I turn to general ethics and examine the history of the virtues, conceptions of virtues and the value of virtues in the lives of moral agents. I describe an advantage and disadvantage of the virtue-based approach to morality.

Chapter 4 – A Critique of Obligation-Based Moral Theories in General Ethics

In this chapter, the critical spotlight is turned on obligation-based moral theories. With regards to general ethics, I critically examine obligation-based moral theories in the form of consequentialism and deontology, and I critique the role of moral obligations, rules and principles[1] within such moral theories.

Chapter 5 – The Origins, Development and Tenets of Virtue Ethics

The focus in this chapter is firmly on virtue ethics, the moral theory that places the virtues at the core of morality. I first describe the origins and development of virtue ethics. Then, I identify three tenets of virtue ethics. I describe both supplementary and strong versions of virtue ethics and as an example of the latter I explore Aristotle's ethics. I examine two central ideas within virtue ethics, namely, moral character and moral education. Finally, I consider the work of Hursthouse[2] concerning virtue ethics' account of action-guidance.

Chapter 6 – Common Objections To Virtue Ethics

I spend this chapter exploring some common objections towards virtue ethics.

Chapter 7 – A Critical Account of Obligation-Based Moral Theories in Nursing Practice

Having objected to obligation-based moral theories in general ethics in Chapter 4, I now focus on the utilization of these theories within nursing practice. First, I present a critical account of obligation-based moral theories in nursing practice. Given these criticisms, I then consider why these theories are so popular in contemporary nursing practice. I outline some examples of the deontic (duty-based) approach in nursing ethics. I then describe the highly influential and popular 'Four Principles'[3] approach to health care ethics and highlight several flaws of obligation-based theories in nursing practice.

Chapter 8 – Virtue-Based Moral Decision-Making in Nursing Practice

In this chapter, I develop a tentative account of the virtue-based approach to moral decision-making in nursing practice. This approach has three features. First, the moral agent cultivates and exercises the moral virtues. Second, the moral agent utilizes judgement in the decision-making process. And third, the moral agent utilizes moral wisdom in the decision-making process. I characterize moral wisdom as a complex idea that consists of (at least) three phenomena. These phenomena are moral perception, moral sensitivity and moral imagination.

Chapter 9 – MacIntyre's Account of the Virtues

Although my account of the virtue-based approach is already reasonably defensible, in this chapter I examine the work of MacIntyre in order to further strengthen its theoretical foundations. I first describe and examine MacIntyre's account of the virtues as set forth in *After Virtue*[4]. I interpret and examine his claims in three sections (S1–S3):

- S1 – The role and importance of MacIntyre's narrative conception of the self in morality;
- S2 – MacIntyre on practices, goods and the virtues;
- S3 – The role and importance of a tradition of enquiry in morality. Objections towards MacIntyre's account are examined.

Chapter 10 – MacIntyre's Account of the Virtues and the Virtue-Based Approach to Moral Decision-Making in Nursing Practice

In this chapter, I apply some of MacIntyre's claims to my account of the virtue-based approach to nursing proposed in Chapter 8.

Chapter 11 – Conclusions

In the final chapter, I summarize my arguments and reiterate some of the problems of the virtue-based approach in nursing practice. Several points for further enquiry and research are noted. I end the book by reiterating some of the merits of the virtue-based approach in nursing practice.

Having provided an outline of each chapter, in the next chapter I shall begin to argue for a virtue-based approach to moral decision-making in contemporary nursing practice.

2
Illness, Narratives and the Value of the Nurse–Patient Relationship

Introduction

An adequate and plausible nursing ethics needs to do much more than merely posit the moral importance of obligation and the moral worth of the consequences of actions and omissions. My central premise is that an adequate nursing ethics needs to begin with a consideration of the *person* who is *ill*. Moreover, such a theory needs to address the moral character traits of nurses; after all, the latter actually *care* for ill persons. Moral obligations do not in themselves care for ill persons. Such deontic concepts require *application* by moral agents. It therefore seems to me crucial that one should examine the sort of nurse one is.

I begin this chapter by exploring several topics that are relevant and important in contemporary nursing practice. These topics are illness and narratives, hospitalization and patients' emotions, the history of the nurse–patient relationship, contemporary views of the nurse–patient relationship and empowerment, the therapeutic or helping nurse–patient relationships, the role of the nurse and definitions of a 'good' nurse. These topics are all crucial to my account of the virtues and the virtue-based approach to moral decision-making in nursing practice.

Illness and narratives

Illness affects humans at any point in the lifespan. 'Illness' is a broad term and in using this term, one is making a value judgement. Illness can be either acute or chronic. It can also be categorized as life-threatening (e.g. malignant cancers), serious (non-life-threatening, e.g. diabetes and arthritis) and minor (e.g. the common cold). However, such reductionist language means that one might not fully understand how a particular illness makes one *feel*. While I have given examples of illness and neatly labelled them, this in no way predicts or explains how a person will respond to or cope with a specific illness. For example, the consensus might well be that the common cold is a 'minor' illness; however, viral infections such as the common cold can cause misery for the sufferer. In this sense then, most, if not all, illness interferes with and causes problems in one's daily living.

During infancy and childhood, children are dependent on others (usually parents or guardians) to care for them and help them to fare well in life. Later in old age the reverse might occur: children may help and care for their parents. During one's life, help and support will often be needed from others, for example, one's spouse, friends and family members. This need might be intensified during periods of physical and mental illness; humans need other humans to help them to fare well during and after illness.

Illness can be a characterizing feature of one's life. This claim is particularly true regarding both physical and mental chronic illness. The extent to which illness becomes part of or takes over one's life depends on several factors, including the causation, symptomatology and prognosis of the illness, and individual personality traits and coping mechanisms. Because of these (and other) factors, illness becomes part of one's life story; in part, illness defines one's life and shapes the sort of life one can live. Importantly, illness is a feature of human life that can be shared with others through, for example, conversation. By sharing these experiences, people can construct a narrative account of their illness, which can help people to find meaning in and make sense of their lives.[1]

Upon reflection, memories of childhood and adult illness come flooding back. Regarding the latter, during illness, I felt bad because of the various symptoms of the actual illness, for example, during a bout of influenza I felt hot, clammy, cold and very tired. Because of previous illness and my knowledge of nursing, I knew that regular fluids and paracetamol would help me to feel better. As a child, my parents would care for me, while nowadays my wife helps me during periods of illness. Reactions to illness are varied and personal. Personally, I feel more upset during illness if I am alone, if no one is around to ask me what I want and no one is present to listen to my moaning. I am not saying that everyone feels like me during illness, but I doubt whether I am alone in feeling like this.

In summary, physical and mental illness and the consequent need for help from others can strike at any point in one's life. One of the few certainties of human life is that one lives each day without knowing when illness will arise; when it does, it becomes a part of one's life that through conversation can be constructed as a narrative.

Hospitalization and patients' emotions

In this section, I will explore some of the many emotions that patients might experience as a result of illness and the effects of hospitalization.

Anxiety

For perhaps the majority of people, feeling anxious is natural during illness; for instance, one might be anxious about the cause and prognosis of the illness. Being hospitalized exacerbates these feelings. In hospital, one is not only anxious about one's well-being, there are also practical issues to worry about. For example, the strange physical environment of an Accident and Emergency (A&E) department or hospital ward and the many new names and faces of health care professionals. Depending upon the severity of one's symptoms, one might be anxious about the potential disabling affects of the illness. Furthermore, being separated from one's spouse and loved ones can also intensify feelings of anxiety. It is not difficult to appreciate why patients often feel anxious during illness and why these feelings might be intensified during hospitalization.

Fear

Fear is an emotion that often coexists with anxiety. People often admit to being frightened at the prospect of being ill. The images that illness conjures up can frighten people, for example, suffering physical pain, emotional distress and needing help from others with one's daily living. Thinking about hospitals and the idea of being hospitalized also scares some people; perhaps this is, in part, because of the public perception of hospitals and the association between hospitals and death and dying. Fear of dying is a natural reaction to life-threatening illness, for example, the fear experienced during an acute myocardial infarction. The experience of illness is always subjective and it is therefore difficult to imagine how such a critical situation might make one feel. Nevertheless, I would suspect that fear of dying would be uppermost in many people's minds during a myocardial infarction and other similar critical illnesses.

Compare the above example with a second one where a person with leukaemia is about to enter hospital for a third course of chemotherapy. This person is frightened because she has vivid memories of earlier distressing experiences of chemotherapy. For instance, she remembers her hair falling out and she cannot forget how painful her mouth was and how tired she was. This person is only too aware of what might occur with the third course of chemotherapy; she is frightened of how she might feel in a week or two and she may well be frightened of dying. In this example, the person remembers the nature of the chemotherapy, especially its side effects. She remembers how physically and emotionally distressed the treatment and side effects will probably make her feel. If we accept the claim that the majority of people wish to lead healthy, independent and valuable lives, then life-threatening illness is likely to create a wide range of emotional responses in the sufferer. For the two people above, the fear of dying from a myocardial infarction and the fear of horrible side effects from chemotherapy are rational emotions to feel.

Powerlessness

Anxiety, fear and all of the features imposed upon one by the dehumanizing process of hospitalization promote feelings of powerlessness. Patients might believe that they have very little input regarding their care; they might feel robbed of all power and control. If patients cannot exert any control over their illness and care, then feelings of powerlessness might naturally develop and these feelings can be deeply upsetting. Feeling powerless is a particular feature of chronic illness. In the words of Pellegrino and Thomasma:

> Sick persons must bare their weaknesses, compromise their dignity, and reveal intimacies of body and mind.[2]

Allowing nurses and other health care professionals access to one's body and mind is necessary in order to survive and recover from illness. However, this can make people feel devoid of power and control; in other words, it can disempower people.

I have briefly considered why patients might feel anxious, frightened and powerless and how these feelings can affect them. Crudely, these negative emotions can be triggered by the illness itself and then intensified owing to the dehumanizing process of hospitalization.

Vulnerability

Patients in hospital are often described as being vulnerable. Feeling vulnerable might arise because one is aware that there is potential to be hurt in the form of physical pain and emotional distress. One's survival might literally be in others' hands. Feelings of anxiety, fear and power-lessness will perhaps contribute to feeling vulnerable. I think that at the core of this notion is a sense of feeling 'wide open to harm'. After all, what could a patient do to prevent harm from befalling him? Patients might be able to prevent or minimize physical harm. However, it is much more difficult if not impossible for a patient to exert any control over the *language* that a nurse might use. In other words, *what* a nurse says and *how* this is phrased is solely under the control of the nurse; patients are not able to control how nurses communicate through language.

Vulnerability and trust

One of the effects that vulnerability has upon patients is that it forces them to trust others. While trust is sometimes described as a voluntary phenomenon, in reality patients have little choice in the matter; for example, Pellegrino and Thomasma[3] claim that patients are forced into trusting clinicians. Irrespective of how qualified nurses are, they are strangers to patients especially during the initial assessment phase. This begs the question: 'Why should patients trust others whom they don't know at all?' In a social setting, few of us would trust a total stranger. But if our choices were limited and death or serious injury was inevitable, then we would be more likely to trust strangers. It is hoped that nurse education ensures that nurses are trained to at least a level of moral and clinical competence if not moral and clinical excellence. Talking to many patients over the years, it strikes me how many assume that all nurses possess certain personal qualities such as kindness, patience and gentleness. A patient will hopefully trust a nurse because of the latter's moral characteristics. However, ultimately, because one is ill and needs help to survive and recover, patients are forced to trust nurses; there is really no alternative unless patients wish to self-discharge. But for most patients, self-discharge is not a viable option, because patients tend to want to survive and recover from illness as quickly as possible. Thus self-discharge would be an irrational[4] act.

As an important aspect of the nurse–patient relationship, trust is a complex notion that has been examined by several nursing scholars.[5] In feminist moral theory, Baier[6] has written widely on trust. She claims that for a moral theory to be adequate and sufficient for both men and women, it needs to include the notions of love and obligation. Crudely, the former will satisfy what most women want in a moral theory, while the latter satisfies what most men want in a moral theory.[7] Baier argues that trust could be the notion that satisfactorily encapsulates both love and obligation. In her view, trusting nurses means relying on their competence; nurses ought to be willing to care for patients who are entrusted to their care. In loving relationships, one trusts another not to harm one, while in relationships founded upon obligation – as nursing is frequently conceived – patients trust nurses to be competent and fulfill their obligations.

Dependence on others

Patients will, depending upon their condition, need to allow nurses direct contact with their bodies. When one is ill and hospitalized, help is needed from nurses (and others) to meet one's needs. Of course, one need not be hospitalized to require help; for example, a person with multiple sclerosis needs twice-daily home visits by community nurses to help meet her needs. Patients are therefore *dependent* on nurses to help them meet their physical and emotional needs; patients *rely* on nurses to relieve their distressing symptoms, promote their independence and enable their recovery. Patients will generally understand that without such necessary interventions their illness might worsen, thus it is appreciated that such interventions are medically necessary. However, as noted earlier, beneath the appearance of voluntariness might lie the fact that patients feel *forced* to trust that nurses are morally and clinically competent.

A brief history of the nurse–patient relationship[8]

Since the middle part of the 20th century the nurse–patient relationship has emerged as central to nursing practice. But at the beginning of the 20th century, patients were viewed and understood as objects of medical and nursing interest. According to Dingwell et al.,[9] nurses were involved in servant–master relationships with medical professionals and had an important role in medical surveillance of the body.[10] There was no meaningful concern with nurse–patient interactions or with personal knowing. Indeed evidence[11] suggests that institutional practices sought to regulate and constrain nurses' interactions with patients. All nurses with the same position and training were considered as equals;[12] all patients were regarded as equal too. Nursing was seen as a 'collective accomplishment'[13] and individual relationships were subsumed within this belief. Personal and professional aspects of nurses were deemed to be mutually exclusive. The personhood of the nurse lay outside her professional role; the personhood of the patient was also deemed to be outside the nurse–patient relationship.

From the 1960s, Armstrong[14] argues, a fundamental change occurred in the development of the nurse–patient relationship. The broadening knowledge base in human psychology and communication theory led to the patient being viewed as a bio-psychosocial being. The idea of a person with physical, psychological and social needs crossed over into developing nursing theories regarding both nurse education and nursing practice. The patient was now seen as a complex subject of nursing care (rather than *just* an object) who needed to be understood. As a result of this change, the humanistic nurse–patient relationship became a central theme in nursing theory.[15] Surveillance was not just a matter of physical identity; it now focused on the patient's bio-psychosocial identity too. Nursing theory and practice, instead of being seen solely in physical or medical terms, developed a holistic[16] person-centred meaning and identity. The organization of nursing work changed from task allocation to individual patient-focused care. As a result, more intimate relationships between nurses and patients could develop.

The nurse–patient relationship in contemporary nursing and the notion of empowerment

The feelings of powerlessness, helplessness, vulnerability and dependence on others for help ensure that the nurse–patient relationship is an unequal one; it is a form of inequality 'paralleled by few other situations in democratic societies'.[17] It is, for many thinkers, the core of nursing and medical practice. For example, according to Pellegrino and Thomasma this relationship is

the moral fulcrum, the Archimedean point at which the balance between self-interest and self-effacement must be struck.[18]

All nursing activities and interventions are enabled through the development, delivery and sustenance of the nurse–patient relationship. However, the inequality that lies at the heart of this relationship contributes towards feelings of powerlessness in patients. Therefore, one of the main issues that needs to be explored in the nurse–patient relationship is the notion of empowerment.

The notion of empowerment is a prominent feature in the current nursing literature.[19] It is possible to explore this notion from several different perspectives and as such, it is difficult to articulate it in simple terms. However, three obvious points emerge from a superficial exploration of the notion of empowerment. First, like many notions that have become popular in health care, it is much more complex than it at first might seem; as noted above, one needs to understand empowerment from several different perspectives such as medicine, psychology, sociology, economics and not least, morality. Second, despite this complexity I shall make two basic claims: the first is that nurses can only empower patients if they themselves have sufficient power and authority; and the second is that nurses should aim to provide a physical and emotional environment that is conducive to patients being able, if they so wish, to make their own decisions. My final point is that an examination of nurses' moral virtues such as respectfulness required to empower patients is neglected in the literature.

Mental illness (or mental ill health[20]) disempowers because one's ability to function on a daily basis is adversely affected by what Barker calls 'problems of living'[21] or the medical model would probably refer to as 'symptoms of mental disorder'. If these features of mental ill health persist then the term 'disabling' is used, and the phrase 'chronic mental illness' is also frequently applied. Clearly, physical illness can also adversely affect one's quality of life. For example, chronic rheumatoid arthritis (CRA) causes pain, deformity and spasticity in the sinovial joints.[22] Living with a chronic illness such as CRA must be difficult; people with CRA usually require anti-inflammatory medications to reduce swelling and promote mobility. The primary focus is on helping people with CRA to meet their needs and retain a sense of independence. People with CRA naturally feel dependent on other people, for example, nurses, doctors and carers to meet their needs. Thus someone with CRA might feel vulnerable and powerless; this feeling might be made worse because they have no control over the course of this chronic progressive illness. Moreover, besides the nature and effects of the illness, the organization and structure of the National Health Service (NHS), for example, primary- and secondary-care institutions, specific treatment processes and legislation such as the Mental Health Act[23] can all add to the feelings of being disempowered.

Latvala et al.[24] described how mental health nurses used three different forms of 'helping' that point to different power dynamics in the nurse–patient relationship. 'Catalytic' helping is described as involving participatory dialogue; mutual collaboration is developed in part because the patient is deemed to have responsible agency. 'Educational' helping is different. Here precedence is given to nurses' knowledge and professionalism, an assumption being that the patient is a responsible recipient; the relationship in this form of helping is driven by the professionalism of the nurse. The third type of helping is termed 'confirmatory', which is based on the assumption that mental ill health arises from a physical cause. Here the patient is a passive recipient of information; the nurse–patient relationship and mutual cooperation is limited by this belief and the hierarchical structure of care services. Even from this brief discussion, it is clear that empowering patients calls for a series of actions and choices that involve nurses making moral judgements. Several factors need to be taken into account including one's values, beliefs, clinical experience and knowledge base. For instance, regarding the first and second factors, a nurse will need to identify and examine her values and beliefs about the cause of a patient's illness and the role that the patient can and should play in their care. (In Chapter 8, I discuss the role of judgement in virtue-based moral decision-making.)

Patients have an individual and unique story to tell concerning their illness; this is the patient's lived experience of the illness. Given the importance of and value attached to the nurse–patient relationship and the benefits of patient-focused care,[25] nurses should allow patients to tell their stories and in doing so, a narrative account of their illness can be told. I imagine that feeling disempowered might arise because the patient is not allowed to tell his or her story; or, perhaps questions are asked, but no one really listens to the patient's story. This might mean that no one learns how the illness is affecting the patient's life. It is easy to understand how patients might feel if they are not given the opportunity to tell their own personal stories.

The medical model and disempowerment

Tilley[26] notes the importance of helping patients and their loved ones to be actively involved in their care. The Department of Health[27] also wish to level the power balance of the nurse–patient relationship and generally, the theme of collaborative care is high on the health care agenda. But, for some thinkers, contemporary mental health nursing practice remains subordinate to the medical model and psychiatry. This view holds that nurses are still the foot soldiers to the generals'[28] (the 'doctors') plans against mental illness. The medical model is clearly focused on clinicians making diagnoses, delivering treatments and identifying and evaluating the outcomes of disease processes and interventions. Epistemologically, the medical model is rooted in empiricism and reductionism. One of the limitations of the medical model is that a patient's lived experience can remain unknown; perhaps this is because the relevant questions are not asked, or no one listens to the patient as he attempts to tell the story of his illness. The medical model emphasizes the disease process and patients' feelings and emotions can remain silent in the benevolent rush to diagnose and treat the disease. However, I am not saying that all or even the majority of clinicians ignore or neglect patients' feelings, that would be far too crude and inaccurate. But the exclusive use of medical language does not promote the identification and examination of patients' feelings and emotions, which are usually seen as subjective and personal notions. Current in vogue initiatives such as patient-centred and holistic nursing care have developed in large part as a reaction against the reductionist approach of empirical medicine. If the medical model is utilized and applied in a singularly scientific manner, then it can hinder the opportunities for patients to tell stories about their illness.

The Tidal Model and empowerment

For several decades, nursing models[29,30] have attempted to adapt and connect general nursing theories to mental health nursing. The Tidal Model,[31] which is a substantial model of mental health nursing practice, is different in the sense that it emerged from a previous study that posed the question: 'What do people need mental health nurses for?' Included within this model is the notion from Peplau[32] concerning the importance of interpersonal interactions. Furthermore, there is recognition that an effective model requires an emphasis on the process of empowerment within the nurse–patient relationship.[33] The Tidal Model proposes that the construction of the patient's lived experience occurs through narrative, which is allowed to develop through the nurse–patient relationship. This model of nursing is an attempt to put the person's lived experience and narrative centre stage, and in doing so, the person can be empowered. The Tidal Model aims to refocus nursing practice on the human needs of people in mental health care. It investigates such notions as personhood, mental distress and the assumption that for many people recovery is possible.

Therapeutic nurse–patient relationships

There is an abundance of literature on the nurse–patient relationship.[34] This relationship is usually termed 'therapeutic', for example, the 'therapeutic' nurse–patient relationship or the 'therapeutic' alliance. The literature discusses several ideas including (a) phases of the nurse–patient relationship, for example, the assessment phase, the working phase and the termination phase, (b) distinctions between social and therapeutic relationships, the latter having distinct aims characterized by the notion of helping another person and (c) communication skills such as empathy and compassion, which it is argued nurses need to develop therapeutic relationships with patients.

How can a therapeutic relationship be defined? Ironbar and Hooper provide one conception:

> The goal, which will take skills and time to achieve, is a therapeutic nurse–client relationship, i.e., one in which the client is enabled to work through his problems, maintain his individuality and to learn from his experiences.[35]

Several texts (see note 9) comment further and list examples of skills that nurses should acquire to develop and sustain therapeutic nurse–patient relationships. These skills include responsiveness, promoting self-esteem, acknowledging the uniqueness of the patient, maintaining confidentiality, making non-judgemental responses, developing trust and empathy and providing support for patients.[36] Yet more thinkers focus on describing processes involved in communication and explain why it is important for nurses to have theoretical knowledge of communication theory. One example of this approach (among many) distinguishes between verbal and non-verbal communication theory.[37] For example, regarding verbal communication, nurses need to think about several aspects of communication including the clarity of one's voice, the brevity of the language, the vocabulary used and meaning, pacing and intonation. Non-verbal communication includes issues such as personal appearance, facial expression, posture, gait, gestures and the use of touch. Skidmore,[38] for one, believes that all of these points are important to facilitate therapeutic relationships. Moreover, he thinks that the notions of reception and understanding are especially vital. 'Reception' refers to full commitment on the part of the nurse to listen carefully to what the patient is saying, while 'understanding' refers to hearing what patients say and then making sense of this information.

Helping relationships

The objectives or ends of a therapeutic relationship are varied and contextual; in mental health nursing, for example, they would include helping a patient into recovery and promoting self-esteem and independent living.[39] In cancer nursing, possible ends might include relieving physical pain, helping a patient to cope with the distress caused by the illness and treatments and helping a patient towards a good death.[40] The literature notes that a 'helping' relationship is an example of a therapeutic relationship and the 'dimensions' of a helping relationship are some-times outlined.[41] For example, to develop helping relationships nurses need to be trustworthy and honest. However, there is no acknowledge-ment that these so-called dimensions are examples of moral virtues. Furthermore, there is no insight into how 'communication skills' and 'dimensions' of communication can be seen from other perspectives, for example, that of morality. Moreover, it is common for the conception of a helping relationship to be articulated in terms of pure communication theory. Human interactions, human responses and the role of moral virtues in developing a helping relationship between nurse and patient are typically ignored. There is a general failure to relate communication, both its theoretical and practice elements, to the moral lives of patients and nurses.

The nurse–patient relationship: Some empirical research findings

There is a wealth of qualitative literature that examines the nurse–patient relationship. For example, a recent three-round Delphi questionnaire study[42] posed the question: 'Describe what you do, think and feel when you build a relationship with a patient?' Seven themes emerged from the 89 points made. In ranking order, these themes were:

1 Getting to know each other;
2 Being open and honest about roles and boundaries;
3 Being friendly towards the client;
4 Recognizing how this person [this client] makes me feel and making sense of this;
5 Showing respect for a person's experience, choices, lifestyle;
6 Developing trust;
7 Giving empathy and sympathy.

All these themes concern either intrapersonal or interpersonal skills or the cultivation of moral virtues. In the same study, participants stated that they based their practice, in part, on moral virtues such as compas-sion, honesty and justice.[43] However, the precise technical term 'moral virtue' meant little to the nurses. But that is unsurprising; why does it matter if compassion, honesty and justice are not understood explicitly as moral virtues? In clinical nursing, I want to see nurses demonstrate moral virtues, for instance, kindness, justice and patience. It does not particularly matter to me whether a nurse is able or unable to articulate a theoretical understanding regarding the meaning of a moral virtue. We should refrain from assuming that there is a correlation between someone's understanding of the moral virtues and how they *actually* act, think and feel. However, perhaps I am being harsh, but I expect greater precision from academic thinkers. If moral virtues are consistently referred to as 'dimensions', then several important issues will remain dormant. Examples of such issues are: the complexity of the virtues, why it is important for nurses to cultivate the virtues, how difficult it can be for nurses to cultivate the virtues and how nurses can use the virtues to make morally good decisions.

Regarding the aforementioned Delphi study, another question asked is: 'What factors might (a) support and (b) restrict this process [building a therapeutic relationship with clients]?' Reponses for (a) included 'taking an interest in people', 'being available to listen to the patient', 'good communication skills' and 'being honest'. All of these responses relate to behaviours, actions and choices that *nurses* had control over. Other responses were given which the respondents believed *patients* had control over, for example, 'a willingness for the client to engage in the relationship' and the 'communication skills of the client'. Responses for (b) included 'lack of respect (or trust) of the client', 'poor communication, e.g., listen too little' and 'poor explanation of the role of the nurse'. These points were recognized as behaviours or qualities within the control of and influenced by the *nurse*. Some of the factors that might restrict the building of a therapeutic relationship and be under the control of the *patient* are 'severe illness', '[clients who are] resistive to involvement' and '[clients] having a bad experience with others'. The role of the moral virtues and the idea of human responsiveness are again seen to be valuable aspects in forming a therapeutic nurse–patient relationship.

The role of the nurse

Describing and clarifying the role of the nurse is complex and it is not conducive to generalization. Contemporary nurses will need to take on several different roles, some of which might be incompatible (just read the list of roles attached to a typical contract of employment to see the variety). When discussing this topic with students, both pre- and post-registration, there is usually some degree of divergence. Specific roles will depend on one's working environment; for example, the roles expected of a theatre nurse will differ from those of a community nurse or mental health nurse working in a forensic unit. However, it might be possible to find some convergence on generic roles that the majority of nurses are expected to meet. Examples of these given in class include 'nurses care for patients' and 'nurses should educate patients about their illnesses'. As noted, several nursing thinkers claim that one important role of the nurse is to utilize intrapersonal and interpersonal skills to facilitate a therapeutic nurse–patient relationship. Another common role articulated in the literature refers to nurses meeting the various physical, psychological, spiritual and social needs of the patient.[44]

In an attempt to clarify nurses' roles, one might be tempted to explicate a single all-important role. What would be the advantage of doing this? It seems to me unnecessary and futile for both individual nurses and the profession to strive for such an objective. Specifying the role of the nurse might provide nursing with a specific identity. For some nurses, depending on the role identified, this might promote the notion of nursing as an independent profession, able to break from the shackles of medicine. But by confining nurses to a discrete role – for example, 'helping patients recover from illness' – it could be argued that nurses' professional and personal autonomy could be threatened. Conversely, a vague role such as 'helping patients recover from illness' could be conceptualized, interpreted and delivered in a wide variety of ways so much so that the role becomes almost meaningless. Again, I am just not sure what the value would be in specifying a single role; I doubt that this endeavour would hinder the development of, for example, one's capacity for independent thought, one's ability to make judgements and the promotion of clinical innovation. All of these qualities are thought important to being an effective professional nurse.[45]

The role of the nurse: Some empirical research findings

Several empirical studies have investigated the role of the nurse and the aims of being a nurse. A recent three-round Delphi questionnaire study[46] revealed some findings about the aims of mental health nurses and their beliefs about the formation of therapeutic nurse–patient relationships. For example, one question was: 'What do you think are the main aims and goals of being a mental health nurse?' This question was posed in round two when 22 mental health nurses participated: 15 females (68%) and 7 males (32%). Eighty-three points were given in response to this question. From these, nine different themes were identified. The most popular themes were:

1 To educate, support and treat people with mental health problems using a range of therapeutic interventions;
2 To utilize skills and knowledge gained through training and life experience to help people who suffer from mental illness;

3 To work with other professionals and outside agencies and the general public to destigmatize mental illness;
4 To see the client as a person, encouraging them to identify their strengths;
5 To develop a rapport and relationship with people.

In this study, the notions of being therapeutic and helpful are expressed in 1 and 2 respectively, 4 points to the idea of providing holistic nursing care, while 5 suggests the importance of an effective nurse–patient relationship.

Another Delphi study supports some of the findings from the one above. This study sought to investigate the required role of the psychiatric-mental health nurse in primary health care.[47] Thirty professionals participated in the study, including community psychiatric nurses, general practitioners, social workers, purchasers and service managers; six participants from each profession were recruited to the study. Following the first and second questionnaires, interviews were held with the professionals. Users of mental health services were then also questioned so that the emergent findings could be verified. The main theme or core category was 'relationships'. It was believed that to provide effective mental health care, nurses needed to develop strong relationships with patients and other professionals. The importance of the nurse–patient relationship, as espoused by thinkers such as Peplau[48] and Altschul[49] was enforced by this Delphi study; in the authors' words:

> There was a view that the value of the nurse-patient relationship was as great, if not greater, than the value of any clinical interventions.[50]

Another recent small-scale study gained qualitative data from users of mental health services. The research question was: 'What do mental health nurses need to be, do, or know?' One of the groups interviewed ($n = 8$) responded with comments that included 'show respect and a genuine interest', demonstrate certain traits such as 'kindness, gentleness and sensitivity' and 'take time to talk and explore difficulties'.[51]

The above three qualitative studies investigated the views of clinical nurses and patients in an effort to describe the reality, not the rhetoric, of nursing for *these* nurses and to ask *these* patients what they wanted from nurses. The emerging themes are not reliable in an empirical sense. For example, if other researchers followed the same methodology, then the findings in other parts of the UK with different participants might well be different. I am not claiming that other nurses and patients from different wards or different geographical locations would *necessarily* concur with the views from these three studies. Although given the literature and the findings from these (and other) studies, it is reasonable to think that there would be some degree of convergence. In sum, the important themes from the three aforementioned studies include (in no particular order):

- Responding to patients as individuals;
- Demonstrating respect towards patients;
- The importance and value of 'relationships', held by some patients to be as great if not greater than the value of other clinical interventions;
- The need to make oneself available to patients, and spend time with them to ask questions, listen to their responses and really hear what they are saying;
- The need for nurses to demonstrate certain traits of character – moral virtues – for example, kindness, patience and honesty.

Barker, Jackson and Stevenson[52] on the essential feature of mental health nursing

Barker et al. recently conducted a modified grounded theory[53] study that broadly investigated the need for and the role of psychiatric nurses. Ninety-two participants including users, family members, friends and mental health professionals took part in a series of focus groups held in two sites in England, two sites in the Republic of Ireland and two sites in Northern Ireland. Theory was generated from participants' statements. Some consensus was provided from both participants and professionals that the 'essential feature of nursing'[54] – the core category – was a complex series of relationships termed 'Knowing you, Knowing me'. Barker prefers to use the terms 'person' or 'people' instead of 'patients' or 'clients'. Three domains of relating were elucidated from this study that 'serve as context-dependent bases for the adoption of differing roles designed to meet the person's needs'.[55] These domains were 'Ordinary Me' (OM), 'Pseudo-Ordinary [or Engineered Me]' (POEM) and 'Professional Me' (PM). OM 'relied on a natural ordinariness' from the nurse, POEM 'involved a more discretely *conscious* presentation of the nurses' "self"', while PM 'is the domain where the nurse did what (s)he considered "best" for the person: the evidence-based domain'.[56] Distinguishing between these domains of relating were four internal dimensions: depth of knowing, power, time and translation.

Depth of knowing

All of the participants stated that nurses *know* people best, i.e., better than medics because of their greater contact time. However, an extensively broad range of knowledge concerning a person might also be superficial in terms of depth of knowledge. The people in this study challenged the belief that too much emotional involvement could be unproductive.[57] Within the OM domain, people wanted nurses to be more intimate and share information about themselves. Often this relationship was one way; as a consequence people lacked motivation to disclose information to nurses considered to be 'blank screens'. While some nurses were comfortable sharing information about themselves within the OM domain, others were not; this was viewed as a burden and emotionally draining.[58]

Power

Regarding the dimension of 'power', differences emerged between the domains of relating. The OM domain involved a sense of caring 'for' someone, while caring 'about' lay within the POEM domain. Barker and Whitehill,[59] while recognizing that caring can include domination by carers, believe that caring 'with' involves active person and nurse collaboration. However, caring 'for' someone 'in such a way as to help them take reasonable risks ... was seen as empowerment'.[60] Within the POEM domain, nurses might hold considerable power but by exercising friendly dispositions, they can win a person's confidence and thus might be able to work on specific therapeutic issues.[61] The nurses in this study did not form friendships but acknowledged being 'friendly':

> I think that you can be friendly without building a friendship ... our role isn't to socialise. There is a goal and we must look for it. I don't see a problem with being friendly to achieve some other goal. (Nurse, group F)[62]

The last part of the above sentence is interesting and to an extent indicates 'a means to an end' approach by the nurse. In some situations, what the nurse says could involve an element of deception or dishonesty, but this might be – as above – justified from the nurse's point of view if a certain goal or outcome is achieved. This relates to the more general theme of needing to be a different nurse to suit individual patients depending upon their needs and expectations. A contemporary conception of the nurse–patient relationship includes the notion of authenticity, i.e., of nurses being authentic and genuine[63] and intimate and empathetic.[64] Arnold,[65] among others, believes that an absence of authenticity leads to a sterile application of communication techniques. However, Aranda and Street[66] claim that problems are created from the view of nurses as authentic. Conflicts arise in nurses who desire to be authentic, and a sense of emotional discomfort and distress afflicts some who feel that in certain complex emotional situations they need to become the sort of person that the patient requires – or, in their words, they need to be 'a chameleon'. These are clearly emotionally turbulent situations and these reflect one of the difficulties for contemporary nurses in balancing their many, sometimes conflicting, roles.

Time

The third dimension was time. Within the OM domain, the use of time was valued as an essential aspect. It was believed that if nurses spent less time with people, then they removed themselves from intimate knowing. Reference was made several times to nurses being unavailable on wards:

> They [the nurses] sit in the office and patients are outside and whether going through distress or whatever, you knock on the door and say can I see somebody. 'You can just wait. You'll be all right. Just go and have a cup of tea.' (Person, group A)[67]

The situation was different within the community setting. Even though the nurses might not spend a lot of time with the person, there were fewer distractions. Community nurses were perceived as having a wider appreciation of families and engaged in more informal and friendly relationships.[68] From the perspective of patients' relatives, the quality of nursing care is affected by several factors and qualities including nurses taking time to get to know the client, working *with* clients and having positive attitudes – even love – for clients.[69]

Some observational literature makes interesting if perhaps surprising reading regarding the amount of time nurses spend in contact with patients. For example, Altschul[70] found that only 8% of psychiatric nurses' time was spent in one-to-one interaction with in-patients. According to Sanson-Fischer et al.[71] only 15.9% of nurses' time was spent on one-to-one therapy, while Martin's[72] study revealed that in-patients spent only 6–12% of their time interacting with staff. In a more recent qualitative study by Jackson and Stevenson,[73] patients stated that they needed time to talk through their problems with nurses. In this study, patients said they valued time more than other interventions utilized in hospital; this supports the finding from the Walker et al. study where patients believed that the value of the nurse–patient relationship was as great, if not greater, than other clinical interventions. According to Hurst and Howard[74], nurses spend more time on administration duties than they do interacting with patients. In the Jackson and Stevenson study, patients stated that they were unlikely to ask nurses for their time and were reluctant to disturb nurses if they were busy. In a recent observational study of 20 staff nurses on three admission wards in a psychiatric hospital, Whittington and McLaughlin[75] found that less than half of the working day (42.7%) was spent in direct patient contact. The study also demonstrated that

> the proportion of work time which was devoted to potentially psychotherapeutic interactions with patients was very small (6.75%).[76]

Translation

Translation was the fourth dimension in the Barker et al. study. Within the OM domain, people and their families wanted nurses to be honest. Truth telling, for example, honestly describing the side effects of medications to people, was valued greatly within these relationships. Nurses were expected to be able to interpret technical jargon and be multilingual, for instance, conversing without difficulty with professional colleagues and also able to converse well with people and their families.

Defining a 'good' nurse

The contemporary definition of a 'good' nurse includes the cultivation of certain personal qualities such as self-awareness, the ability to reflect about practices including self-reflection and the demonstration of interpersonal skills.[77] In a recent Delphi study,[78] one question was: 'What is it to be a 'good' mental health nurse?' Eighteen respondents (81.8%) stated that this was concerned with (a) practical skills, (b) clinical experience and (c) moral qualities. No one suggested that the development of competent practical skills was related to how long one had been a nurse. Two of the responses were: 'Moral qualities and moral experience affects how a nurse delivers these practical skills, as it is about who she [the nurse] is as a person' and 'It is a mixture of both but mainly it is the moral qualities and experience, To be honest and respectful of the client.' The latter respondent made the point that knowledge and experience gained in practice and used to benefit the patient was, therefore, a moral 'thing'; I would prefer the term 'enterprise', but the point is well made and understood.

Three respondents stated that both practical skills and moral qualities were important to being a good nurse; however, a third factor 'general life experiences' was necessary too. For example:

> Skills, experience and general life experiences would be my main positive aspect, feeling you could offer people help from known experiences. Though moral qualities would still be an important issue which would help me examine, [and] improve my standards of care.[79]

In the above quote, the respondent appears to believe that moral qualities include intrapersonal skills such as self-reflection and that these qualities can be utilized to promote one's own caring abilities or competence. Finally one respondent stated that being a good mental health nurse concerned *only* the importance of moral qualities. She seemed to indicate the value of making a connection with a patient and generally the value of holistic nursing care. In her words: 'A good nurse is someone who can identify with patients and regard them as people in their own right.'

Empirical research findings suggest that patients have their own views regarding what constitutes 'good-' or 'high-'quality nursing care. One small-scale study[80] involved interviewing 24 patients with mental health problems from two admission wards in a psychiatric hospital. Qualitative analysis revealed 239 indicators of high- and low-quality nursing care, which the authors categorized into six main themes. One theme was 'communicating caring' and this comprised three subthemes, 'being available', 'listening' and 'actions explained'. Under 'being available', the responses indicated that the patients valued the nurses as caring if they made themselves available to the patients. Nurses' actions that were particularly appreciated by the patients included setting time aside to be with patients, and nurses' attempts to understand patients' problems. Under 'listening' several patients said that it was more important to them that nurses listened to their conversations than what the nurses actually said in response. Some negative experiences of not being listened to were described in the interviews. One patient remarked:

> There's one nurse, if she sits and talks to you she is always looking around to see if anything is happening ... she's not really bothered with what I'm saying and will come up with any answer just to shut me up.[81]

Theme six was termed 'nurses' attributes'. In this theme, the patients described the personal qualities, which they believed contributed to high-quality nursing care. Examples of these traits were 'being caring', 'friendliness', 'kindness', 'patience' and 'tolerance'. In this study, patients with mental health problems were able to sense and perceive virtuous care, that is, care motivated and exercised from moral virtues such as kindness and patience.

Conclusions

This chapter has described and examined several areas of nursing practice that help to lay the foundations for the remainder of this book. Several conclusions can be drawn from the preceding discussion. First, illness can affect one at any point in the lifespan. Illness becomes part of the person; it is therefore a personal phenomenon. Second, illness whether it is life threatening or not causes a range of emotional responses in the person including feelings of anxiety, fear, helplessness, powerlessness and vulnerability. These feelings can be intensified with admission to hospital. Ultimately, when one is hospitalized one is dependent upon help from others including nurses to fare well during and after illness. Third, there seems to be a relationship between human vulnerability caused by illness and human dependence on others for help. MacIntyre[82] points out that this relationship has been ignored in moral philosophy. I would also suggest that this relationship has been largely ignored in much of the nursing ethics literature.

The helping nurse–patient relationship is held by patients to be extremely valuable, as valuable, if not *more* valuable, than other clinical interventions. It seems to me that this kind of helping relationship is only achievable if nurses make themselves available to patients, spend sufficient time with patients, allow patients to tell their stories and listen to patients' stories. However, the literature suggests that nurses are spending most of their time doing administrative tasks, with only a small proportion of their time spent in direct contact with patients.

The theoretical and empirical literature reviewed agrees on certain characteristics of a therapeutic nurse–patient relationship. These include the idea that this relationship should be patient-centred and mutually collaborative. The role of the nurse is a complex topic, one not amenable to assumptions and gross generalization. From a review of the theoretical and qualitative literature and from my own clinical and teaching experiences, it is possible to identify several areas of convergence. Broadly these include the idea that nurses should help the patient to survive, recover and be independent. Being a 'good' nurse and providing 'high-'quality care from the perspectives of nurses', patients' and patients' relatives centres on the delivery of several personal attributes, qualities or skills. These include the need for nurses to: develop and demonstrate good verbal and non-verbal communication skills; be friendly towards patients, treat patients with respect and meet patients' individual physical and non-physical needs (holistic nursing care); and finally, demonstrate personal qualities or 'dimensions' such as trustworthiness, honesty, patience and kindness. The latter are more accurately understood as examples of moral virtues. Despite not framing them as 'moral virtues', the nursing literature suggests that the virtues are crucial to developing helping relationships, being a 'good' nurse and to the end of delivering 'high-'quality care.

Having clearly identified examples of the moral virtues and highlighted their importance within the helping nurse–patient relationship, I turn to general ethics and examine the moral virtues in more detail in Chapter 3.

3
The Virtues in General Ethics

Introduction

In the previous chapter, I highlighted the importance of the moral virtues in the development of a helping nurse–patient relationship. In this chapter, I turn to general ethics and take this discussion further. The discussion of the virtues is confined to general ethics to lay some of the theoretical foundations for the remainder of this book. In this chapter, I focus on the place of the virtues in the history of philosophy, I attempt to define virtues and vices, I consider why the virtues are valuable in human lives and I briefly note an advantage and disadvantage of the virtue-based approach to morality.

On 'faring well'

I believe that autonomous persons with decision-making capacity usually want their needs to be met and interests promoted. Physical needs must be met or illness will occur and people want their emotional and social needs met so that their lives possess a certain level of quality; generally, lives are enriched and people fare well if their needs are met. Should I say more about the notion of a life faring well? In this book, one's life goes well if needs are met and interests promoted and the arbiter of this state of affairs is the person concerned. For instance, if I wanted to form good long-lasting friendships with other people and this did not happen, then my life – in terms of this one desire – has not fared well; at least it has fared less well than I desired it would. Or suppose that I wanted to become financially wealthy and despite my best efforts this did not occur. I might judge that my life has not fared well in terms of this one (important) desire. Other human desires, aims and life plans include wanting to achieve certain career aspirations, wanting to travel the world, wanting to develop personal qualities such as self-confidence, and wanting to be healthy. Whenever these objectives are not successfully met and there is, therefore, a gulf between reality and one's desires, it is possible that one might judge that one's life has not fared as well as one had hoped.

The virtues in the history of philosophy

Ancient Greek philosophy provides an early account of the role of the virtues in human lives, understood in terms of human nature, the good life for humans and the notion of human flourishing.[1] However, when examining Plato and Aristotle's ethics it should be remembered that for the ancient Greeks, ethics and politics were deeply interconnected, the primary objective being to form and maintain just states. Thus the idea of virtue was understood in terms of how it could help men to protect their states.

In *The Nicomachean Ethics*, Aristotle's central question was 'What is the good life for man?' Crudely, his response was that the good life for man consisted in living the life of virtue according to reason and desires (I discuss Aristotle's ethics in more detail in Chapter 5). With the monotheism of Christianity, the virtues were neglected and God was seen as a lawgiver. According to God, righteous living meant obedience to the divine commandments. The Christian thinker, St. Augustine, distrusted reason; instead, he held that to be morally good one needed to subordinate oneself to the will of God. Thus the theological virtues – faith, hope, charity and obedience – held a central place in Divine Law. In the medieval period, Aquinas devoted a large part of *Summa Theologiae*[2] to the virtues. The Enlightenment saw the rise of Reason and a return to secular ethics. In the 17th century, Hobbes[3] believed that glory and profit were the only human motives.[4] However, the virtues of sympathy and benevolence were at the core of Hume's ethics. And although Kant is held to be one of the founders of deontology, he argued in 'The doctrine of virtue'[5] that persons had strict (perfect) duties to cultivate the virtues.[6] Kant's Moral Law replaced Divine Law and the pivotal question in moral philosophy became 'What is the right thing to do?' The broad aim of the Moral Law was to produce a system of moral rules so that individuals, who were obliged to follow these rules, could know which actions were right and wrong. Thus, modern moral philosophers as a result of going in a different direction from the ancient Greeks, developed theories of obligation, for example,

Kantianism and utilitarianism, instead of theories of virtue. While this account is brief and incomplete because it treats over 2000 years of human history in less than a page, it is nevertheless accurate and representative of the development of obligation-based moral theories.[7]

What is a virtue?

Aristotle on virtue

In Book two of *The Nicomachean Ethics*, Aristotle states that the soul consists of three kinds of things: passions, faculties and states of character. Aristotle believed that virtue is neither passions nor faculties; 'All that remains is that they [the virtues] should be *states of character*'.[8] Aristotle distinguished between moral and intellectual virtue. The latter were taught through instruction and were divided into scientific knowledge (*episteme*), intelligence (*nous*), technical skill (*techne*), wisdom (*sophia*) and practical wisdom (*phronesis*). Conversely, moral virtue was acquired through exercising the virtue, 'moral virtue comes about as a result of habit'.[9] The word 'habit[ual]' is crucial; take honesty as an example, someone who is honest on *certain* occasions – perhaps when it is convenient to be so – does not possess the virtue of honesty. In the Aristotelian view, the honest person is *always* honest. For Aristotle, the actions of a virtuous person spring from a steady unchangeable character.

I discuss Aristotle's ethics in more depth in Chapter 5. For now, I shall say that Aristotle believed that the virtuous person would fare better in life than the non-virtuous person.

Are the virtues types of knowledge?

In *Meno*[10], Plato discusses the idea that virtue is knowledge. In ancient Greece, to possess knowledge was to be virtuous; in other words, knowledge of the good life *made* a man good. But, like Aristotle, Plato held that only certain people – in fact, only Athenian gentlemen, women were excluded – could achieve the status of virtue. I shall discuss the idea that virtue is knowledge in more detail. While I have not yet examined the nature of specific virtues, I cite examples to make this debate more fruitful.

A simple dictionary definition of the word 'knowledge' is 'awareness or familiarity gained by experience (of a person, fact, or thing)'.[11] Are virtues such as courage and justice types of knowledge? Could a virtue such as compassion be knowledge? It is clear that contradictions spring from the claim that virtue is knowledge. For instance, Sam displays courage when she rescues the child from the path of the oncoming car. During the rescue, Sam's leg is injured. In the light of her injury, it might be thought that Sam lacked wisdom. If this is accepted, then Sam possessed *and* lacked virtue, i.e., she possessed the moral virtue of courage but lacked the intellectual virtue of wisdom. However in trying to rescue the child, Sam was aware that she could get hurt. Action in the face of possible danger partly characterizes courage. It is not easy to save a child's life when serious harm to oneself might occur. Realizing the potential for harm makes the deed even more admirable. Afterwards Sam might act with great humility, responding to others' compliments with 'Oh, I didn't have time to think ... anyone would have done the same ... I'm not courageous.' But underestimating the measure of her act and reflecting modestly about the deed are themselves admirable personal qualities. Now, consider justice as a virtue. To act justly, one needs to know what it means to be just. In this sense, the notion of having knowledge is a necessary condition of being a virtuous (i.e., just) person. Is there a connection between having knowledge of a specific virtue and being virtuous? Does such knowledge encourage and promote self-reflection and a deeper level of thinking? It is of course entirely possible for someone to have a deep knowledge of, for example, the virtue of justice and yet that person is unjust and this obvious point applies to all virtues. The reverse is also true, i.e., a just man might have never read any literature on the virtue of justice. These questions remind me about some of my students' assumptions regarding teachers of nursing ethics. During teaching and learning sessions, it has transpired that some students assume that because I teach ethics, I must therefore be a moral person. Having knowledge of any discipline is something that can be admired. However, it is plainly untrue to suggest that having a theoretical understanding of ethics necessarily means that the possessor is a moral person. It is as difficult for me to be moral than it is for others including novice students of nursing who are beginning to learn about the complexities of ethics.

Perhaps the claim that virtue is knowledge should be understood in terms of having wisdom or being a wise person. It is commonly supposed that people become wise through experience. But experiences are personal. Furthermore, personal interpretation lies at the core of understanding experiences and learning from them. Even if two people could undergo the same experience, they will perceive elements of the situation differently, interpret the situation in different ways, focus on different things and as such, their learning will be dissimilar. Merely having many experiences does not necessarily make someone wise.

I reject the use of the singular 'virtue' because I am referring to character *traits*. Therefore, I cannot accept the idea that 'virtue' is knowledge in the formal sense of the word. However, I accept that acting virtuously requires people to possess forms of knowledge gained through familiarity and comprehension of previous experiences.

The contemporary meaning of the term 'virtue'

Two uses of the word 'virtue' can be readily distinguished. First, when it is used as a noun, virtue can mean 'advantages' or 'strengths' as in 'this system has the following virtues.' Second, 'virtuous' may be used as an adjective in relation to persons, for example, 'Carol is a virtuous woman'. Both usages provide positive and complimentary descriptions, which imply praiseworthiness; 'virtue' is not used in a negative sense.

Assumptions about virtues and goodness

At this point, I will briefly address one of the common criticisms of the virtues, namely that it is assumed that the virtues are good. The main objection is that virtue ethics – in short, the moral theory that places the virtues at the core of morality – is therefore circular in nature, i.e., that by being virtuous – for example, honest – one is a morally good person, but to be morally 'good' one needs to be virtuous. While this is one of the traditional criticisms levelled at virtue ethics, it does not fatally undermine the coherence of it. The term 'virtue' derives from the ancient Greek word '*arête*' and means 'an excellence of character'.[12] Since ancient Greece, the term 'virtue' has been used to mean good or excellent character traits. This usage is widely accepted. The moral philosophies of Socrates, Plato and Aristotle, not to mention several influential contemporary virtue ethicists[13] defend this usage and counter the circular argument criticism.

Another way of explaining the supposed assumption concerning the goodness of virtues is to return to the earlier debate on knowledge. There appears to be a relationship between on the one hand the idea that knowledge and virtue are synonymous and on the other hand, the common view concerning the positive value of knowledge *per se*. It seems to me that many people place a high value on the idea of 'knowledge', of being 'knowledgeable' and of 'knowing' something about themselves, others or the external world. It is often said that having knowledge is a 'good' thing and we tend to perceive individuals who lack knowledge to be 'inferior' in some sense. Moreover, in contemporary health care ethics the relationship between possessing knowledge and being autonomous is well established, for example, the notion of making informed decisions. It is important to think about the purpose and uses of knowledge and therefore whether knowledge is intrinsically or instrumentally valuable, i.e., is knowledge valuable for its own sake or for what it might be used for? It seems to me that many of us admire people whom we perceive to be knowledgeable; it also seems to me that we sometimes envy those whom we perceive to be 'clever'. I accept the claim that typically people believe that knowledge *per se* is a good thing and that it is therefore of value. If this is true and if there is a connection between the value of knowledge and the wisdom required to be virtuous, then it might lead to the belief that the virtues are also a good and therefore should be cultivated.

Virtues or vices?

Aristotle's conception of a virtue fails to distinguish virtues from vices because the latter are also character traits manifested in habitual action. Pincoffs provides one account of how to resolve this problem. He claims that the virtues and vices should be thought of as qualities that people think about in deciding whether someone should be avoided or sought. He writes:

> Some sorts of person we prefer; others we avoid ... The properties on our list can serve as reasons for preference or avoidance.[14]

Regarding the vices, most people would probably wish to avoid meeting others who are, for instance, cruel, callous, mean or dishonest. Such character traits are not admirable either in oneself or in others, thus people who cultivate and exercise the vices should not be worthy of praise or admiration.

Is it possible to provide a complete list of virtues?

There are numerous moral virtues and naturally, it is difficult to be accurate about the exact number. Just think for a moment about the wide range of complimentary adjectives at our disposal. I think that many of these qualify as moral virtues, for instance, an *honest* person, a *kind* person, a *patient* person and a *tolerant* person. The virtues are sometimes sub-divided in an attempt, I think, to make these traits easier to remember, understand and apply in concrete situations. For example, compassion, honesty, benevolence and patience are among the so-called other-regarding virtues. Justice and fairness are classed as social or civic virtues. Other perhaps less widely acknowledged virtues include assertiveness, tolerance and temperance. The latter do not appear to be categorized. The literature does not speculate on the number of possible virtues and it is the same for alternative moral theories. For example, there is no preoccupation with the 'total' number of moral principles or the total number of moral rights. Rachels provides a list of common virtues.[15] However, one needs to note that a list merely functions to provide examples of virtues and as a result, any list will be incomplete. If someone presented to me a list of 25 moral virtues and argued that it was the complete definitive list, I might respond by saying, 'Oh, this list is quite comprehensive, but what about respectfulness ... or trustworthiness?' An amended list of 27 (the 25 on the list, plus respectfulness and trustworthiness) moral virtues might then be presented. But later on someone else gazes at the list and says 'Oh, it's a good list but what about courage?' And of course this process would continue. I disagree with those who allege that the inability to produce a complete list of virtues is objectionable. Instead it serves to remind us just how complex human lives and morality are. Furthermore, it ensures that reflection on possible candidates for the status of virtues is not only possible, but remains an exercise in human intellect that should be encouraged and admired. In short, it seems to me that believing that lists of virtues are 'complete' means that opportunities for philosophizing about morality and the moral character of persons are lost.

What might determine important virtues?

Virtues and roles

Peoples' lives consist of many diverse roles. It therefore seems sensible to suggest that different virtues will need to be cultivated if one wishes to be successful. Rachels[16] gives two examples, an auto mechanic and a teacher. He believes that an auto mechanic should be honest, conscientious and skilful, while a teacher should be articulate, patient and knowledgeable. Take a lawyer as another example. I would like my lawyer to be intelligent, articulate and courageous. By exercising these traits, my lawyer could act well as my advocate and promote and safeguard my legal rights (note, however, that I might also wish my lawyer to be deceitful or at least not always honest). It can be seen that the cultivation of the virtues depends upon one's roles.

Is a single set of virtues desirable for all persons?

Given the above, it would seem that the answer here is in the negative. Because there are so many contrasting roles, a wide range of different virtues will be required for people to live morally good lives. Is it useful to think in terms of 'the good person'? This might imply that everyone evolves from the same mould. Nietzsche for one challenged this claim. In rejecting the assumption that only one form of human goodness exists, he said:

> How naïve it is altogether to say: 'Man *ought* to be such-and-such!' Reality shows us an enchanting wealth of types, the abundance of a lavish play change of forms – and some wretched loafer of a moralist comments: 'No! Man ought to be different'. He even knows what man should be like, this wretched bigot and prig: he paints himself on the wall and exclaims, 'Ecce Homo!'[17]

Nietzsche is not readily recognized as a philosopher interested in the virtues. However, the above quotation illustrates that he believed that many forms of human goodness exist. On his view, the virtues would differ from person to person depending on, for example, one's professional and social roles. Historical eras need also to be taken into account as norms of behaviour are interpreted within the context of history. For example, qualities in two women in different periods of history may both (in different ways) be virtuous and admirable. According to Rachels:

> A Victorian woman who would never expose a knee in public and a modern woman on a bathing-beach have different standards of modesty. And yet all may be admirable in their own ways.[18]

Do the virtues differ within different societies?

The short answer is in the affirmative, however much depends on the kinds of practices,[19] institutions and values deemed permissible and sustained in particular societies. In other words, the answer to this question depends in part on the sorts of lives humans are able to live within different societies. Different societies play an important part in grounding and influencing the cultivation of virtues. A question worth asking therefore is, 'do all people need some virtues irrespective of the era?' On this, Aristotle remarked:

> One may observe in one's travels to distant countries the feelings of recognition and affiliation that link every human being to every other human being.[20]

Here, Aristotle is suggesting the universality of (at least) some virtues. Certain essential human needs, for example, physiological needs such as respiration and eating and drinking remain the same irrespective of one's culture. Are moral virtues important in satisfying human needs? It might at first appear that with regard to physiological needs, moral virtues are only of limited use (I would argue that intellectual virtues such as practical wisdom are much more important in meeting physical needs). In satisfying non-physical needs such as the need to form friendships, it is plausible to suggest that moral virtues such as trustworthiness, honesty and loyalty are, irrespective of one's cultural background, important in meeting these needs.

What is a virtue? Revisited

I return now to the question, what is a virtue? According to contemporary moral philosophers,[21] moral virtues are character traits that dispose their possessor to habitually act, think and feel in certain ways. Rachels, for example, believes that a virtue is 'a trait of character, manifested in habitual action that it is good for a person to have'.[22] The virtues form part of one's character; they are an internal part of one's identity. Moral obligations are external to the person; social constructs such as obligations are imposed on people from the outside world, for example, professional obligations from the Nursing and Midwifery Council[23] and legal obligations derived from statutory and common law. External constructs such as obligations need to be conceived, interpreted and applied by people, hence they are not necessarily compatible with the kind of person one is. I mentioned above that the virtues dispose people to act, think and feel in certain ways. To be more specific and following Aristotle, the virtues are *excellences* of character. Thus the moral virtues are morally excellent character traits. Cultivating and exercising the moral virtues is instrumental to leading morally good lives. Exercising the moral virtues tends to help people to fare well in life and helps others fare well too. However, I stress that I am talking about faring well in moral terms, for example, being dishonest might help one to become financially wealthy, but this kind of life is not a morally good life. Cultivating the moral virtues will help one to act, think and feel in morally excellent ways. I would add that the virtues should be regarded as morally admirable traits of character.[24] People who exercise moral virtues deserve to be praised and admired because of the moral excellence of their deeds, thoughts and feelings and because it can be extremely difficult to cultivate the virtues. This conception of a moral virtue is used throughout the remainder of this book, although it is amended in Chapter 9 in the light of MacIntyre's claims about internal goods and the notion of a practice.

Why should the virtues be valued?

The examples of honesty and kindness

I have stated that the moral virtues are to be understood as morally excellent character traits that help people to lead morally good lives and deserve praise and admiration from others. It seems to me that an obvious question is 'What reasons are there for *not* valuing the virtues?' As noted earlier, the virtues might not be valued because it is not easy to be habitually virtuous; one only needs to think about an other-regarding virtue such as generosity to appreciate this point. If one does not wish to lead a completely altruistic life, then it is clear that one might not immediately (if at all) understand the value of the virtues especially other-regarding virtues. Furthermore, valuing the virtues will also depend upon the particular virtue in question. Take the virtue of honesty as an example. If I exercise the virtue of honesty, i.e., do honest deeds and think and feel in honest ways, then I will successfully form and maintain mutually beneficial friendships. Of course, it is assumed here that the honest person would also be selfless and loyal. In other words, if I cultivate one virtue – in this case honesty – I would necessarily cultivate other virtues. This view is based on the idea that the person who cultivates the virtue of honesty does so after deep reflection and deliberation. Such a person truly wants to become virtuous, because she is aware of how exercising the virtues can positively affect the flourishing of other people and herself. Given this claim, it does seem strange if not self-defeating that this person would decide to only cultivate a single virtue.

Regarding why[25] it is good to cultivate the virtues, typically humans are rational and social creatures who prefer to live in communities. To interact with each other successfully, virtues such as honesty, justice and loyalty are important so long as humans wish to get on well together. What might happen if people cultivated the vices of dishonesty, injustice and disloyalty? We would be less inclined to trust people who were dishonest and we would be more inclined to live in isolation or in smaller groups if we thought people were dishonest and we did not trust them. Perhaps in time, communities would fragment and disintegrate and close relationships would be unsustainable. Imagine the effects on communities if people tended to be dishonest *and* unjust *and* disloyal? As noted, peoples' roles differ and we have different interests and needs. A wide range of virtues are of value in successfully achieving these roles and ends.

As I think the above discussion shows, it is not easy to provide a simple answer to the question 'Why should the virtues be valued?' In an effort to demonstrate the value of the virtues, I will look at a second example, that of kindness. Robert is a charity worker in Africa, helping to care for people who are sick and dying. He is kind towards others. He believes that being kind is crucial to his role because he can see that those whom he cares about are helped through his acts and feelings of kindness. Importantly, Robert also intuitively believes that the people whom he helps *feel* his kindness. Robert works consistently hard to be kind towards others. By acting, thinking and feeling kindly, Robert carries out his role well and others are helped through his kindness. This example is limited to one other-regarding virtue, namely, kindness and it could be accused of oversimplifying the reality of charity work. However, it serves to show how the virtues are important in human lives; how, in this scenario, Robert's kindness helped others to fare better in life and how it helped him to do well too.[26] This example also shows how exercising the moral virtues especially other-regarding virtues such as kindness, is particularly important when working with people who are helpless and vulnerable (as noted in Chapter 2).

The more difficult examples of chastity and temperance

Irrespective of the problems noted, the virtues of honesty and kindness are clear-cut examples of virtues. Honesty and kindness are examples of traits that most people view as positive qualities, qualities that deserve one's admiration. However, when the virtue in question relates to behaviour that is not widely valued, then the virtue requires scrutinizing. According to Benn, chastity is such a 'virtue'. Benn asks 'What is so admirable about chastity?'[27] He is sceptical that appealing to this virtue can provide plausible reasons for sexual restraint. Another example is temperance, a trait highly valued by Aristotle. For some people, moderating their behaviour, for example, curtailing their alcohol consumption or reducing their dietary intake are extremely difficult things to do. This discussion leads to the question 'Which traits of character are virtues and which are not?' This is an important question because the charge of moral relativism looms large if this question is not satisfactorily resolved (this question is addressed in Chapter 5).

Advantages of the virtue-based approach to morality

Crudely, virtue ethics is the moral theory that makes the virtues central to morality. In this section, I examine the moral force of virtue and vice terms. (In Chapter 5, I examine virtue ethics' rich account of moral motivation and moral character, and then in Chapter 8, I develop an account of the virtue-based approach to moral decision-making in nursing practice.)

Action-guidance from virtue and vice terms

One of the central tenets of a moral theory is that it should provide adequate action-guidance for moral agents. In moral dilemmas, an adequate moral theory should help a person to know what ought to be done. With regard to action-guidance, Hursthouse[28] believes that it is important to think about the broad range of vice terms to be found within the vocabulary of the virtues and vices; indeed she believes that in comparison the list of virtues is relatively short. Not only is the list of vices long, these terms are also remarkably useful to one's conduct. According to Hursthouse, virtue terms such as 'honest', 'fair', 'kind' and 'patient', and the opposite vice terms 'dishonest', 'unfair', 'unkind' (or 'cruel') and 'impatience' provide people with greater explanatory force compared with obligations and deontic terms (I discuss this point in relation to the work of nurses in more depth in Chapter 7). Anscombe heavily influences Hursthouse's view on this point. Anscombe believes that instead of using deontic terms 'it would be a great improvement if, instead of "morally wrong" one always named a genus such as "untruthful", "unchaste", "unjust" ... the answer would sometimes be clear at once'.[29] Hursthouse believes that people can gain a lot of 'invaluable action guidance ... from avoiding courses of action that are irresponsible, feckless ... harsh ... feeble ... self-indulgent'.[30] Simply put, the claim is that we can gain a lot of action-guidance by thinking hard about the virtue and vice terms and the sorts of deeds expected of someone who exercises specific virtues or vices. For example, suppose I wonder whether I can justify lying to Adam. I can get a clearer idea of how I ought to act by considering whether the range of behaviours open to me are honest, fair or hurtful rather than by asking whether the behaviours are right, wrong, ethical or unethical. Actually, how much action-guidance is forthcoming from the prescription, 'do what is ethical'? How can this crude prescription help me when I find myself in a morally complex situation and I simply do not know what I should do? Benn suggests that virtue and vice terms such as kind and dishonest carry 'rhetorical resonance' that can positively affect one's behaviour. So, for example, upon hearing 'you should do what the *kind* agent would do' I get a sense of the range of acts, thoughts and feelings that kind persons are known for. Perhaps upon deeper thinking, I become more aware of the meaning of 'being kind'. Benn believes that 'words like *dishonest* play a more central role in everyday moral talk than words like *wrong*'.[31] I agree with this claim. Many parents use the virtue and vice terms with their children on a regular basis. It seems to me that as one develops into adulthood, words such as 'fair' and 'kind' are replaced with deontic language especially the central concepts of 'right' and 'wrong'. While Benn holds that the idea of right and wrong action should not be dispensed with, he also believes that the use of virtue and vice terms can be very helpful by providing a rich sense of action-guidance.

Problems with the virtues

Identifying the virtues[32]

In this section, I briefly note the problem of identifying the virtues. Disagreement exists on which character traits are virtues. For example, one person compiling a list of virtues might believe that honesty, patience and tolerance are virtues. Another person may disagree, instead favouring compassion and integrity. However, I am sceptical that a person who advocates the virtue-based approach to morality would, on the one hand, defend honesty and on the other hand reject compassion. On my view, a virtue is a character trait habitually performed that disposes one to act, think and feel in morally excellent ways. People who exercise the virtues deserve praise and admiration and the fact that there are so many plausible virtues is not sufficient reason to claim that these traits are not *all* virtues.

Instead of the above claim, perhaps a more powerful claim is that there *are* only *several* virtues. This view runs counter to the claim that I made earlier in this chapter that numerous different virtues exist. For instance, the above claim is that *only* honesty, patience and tolerance *are* virtues, therefore ruling out other candidates such as kindness. I reject this claim. It seems to me implausible to believe that the moral life can be exhausted by reference to three character traits. One who suggests that there are only three virtues (or fewer) needs to respond to several questions including 'How can humans live morally good lives without being *just*?' In other words, without the virtue of justice is it possible to be morally good and if so, how? If the response to this question is affirmative, then one must be committed to a view of moral goodness that excludes the common idea that moral goodness involves being a just and fair person.

Conclusions

While extremely difficult, cultivating the moral virtues and habitually exercising them will help one to act, think and feel in morally excellent ways. The virtues should be regarded as morally admirable traits of character, and people who exercise the virtues ought to be praised and admired because of the moral excellence of their deeds, thoughts and feelings. In sum, cultivating the moral virtues helps moral agents to lead successful, morally good lives. Advantages of the virtue-based approach to morality include the rich and highly textured degree of action-guidance derivable from the virtue and vice terms. However, problems with this approach include the supposed difficulty in identifying the virtues.

In Chapter 4, I critically examine the role of moral obligations in morality and critique the moral theories of consequentialism and deontology.

4
A Critique of Obligation-Based Moral Theories in General Ethics

Introduction

I have identified that moral virtues such as honesty and kindness are extremely important to the development and sustenance of a helping nurse–patient relationship. Moreover, what patients and patients' relatives call 'high-' quality nursing care, I would call 'virtuous' nursing care. In the previous chapter, I explored the notion of a virtue and attempted to explain why the moral virtues are valuable in human lives. This chapter is devoted to a critical examination of the role of moral obligations and their underpinning moral theories in general ethics. This chapter is necessary because obligation-based moral theories such as consequentialism and deontology are popular theories not just in general ethics but nursing ethics too. I want to explore the merits and criticisms of these deontic moral theories. I first outline the moral theory known as consequentialism, focusing to a large degree on act-consequentialism. Then, deontology is put under the critical spotlight. In this chapter, the broad aim is to show that the standard objections to these deontic theories outweigh their supposed merits.

Characterizing obligation-based moral theories

Obligation-based[1] moral (or ethical[2]) theories can be characterized, fairly accurately, as theories that emphasize the role of moral obligations, moral rules or moral principles in morality. Crudely, obligation-based theorists hold that the role of moral obligations is crucial in morality; they believe that moral obligations are central to ethics and that acting from obligation ensures morally right conduct. Obligation-based theories hold that persons are obliged to do certain things or behave in certain ways towards others; that people owe obligations towards each other.[3] Anscombe believed that modern moral philosophy, i.e., utilitarianism and Kantianism[4] is bound up with obligation and duty simply because of the history of moral philosophy. In both the moral philosophy and applied ethics literature, the two predominant types of obligation-based moral theories are consequentialism (including utilitarianism) and deontology. Both types of theory focus upon actions and omissions, and advocates of these theories tend to ask questions that represent this focus, for example: 'What ought I to do?', 'What is the right course of action?' and 'Of these two (or more) choices, which one is the best?'

Consequentialism

Consequentialists can be described as 'forward looking' theorists because they believe that the events after an act are what characterize the morality of the act. Consequentialists argue that what make right acts right (and wrong acts wrong) are the act's consequences, outcomes or results.[5] Typically, consequentialist theories take the form: 'Act x is right if x produces good consequences.' Many consequentialists go further and insist that 'good' is insufficient; the consequences of an act have to be the *best* among a range of possibilities, in other words, the utility of the act has to be maximized.

Act-consequentialism

An example of a consequentialist moral theory is act-consequentialism,[6] which according to Frey holds 'that an act is right if its consequences are at least as good as those of any alternative'.[7] This theory is consequentialist because it views the rightness and wrongness of acts in terms of their actual consequences. It is worth noting two criticisms, even at this early point. First, this formulation ignores many other morally important features, for example, intentions and motives. And second, doubt is raised on the question of how one can *know* the actual consequences of an act. In response to the latter criticism, two things can be said. First, it is true to claim that people cannot see into the future and predict the consequences of an act. But consequentialists allege that experience and wisdom can provide some general guidelines regarding the sorts of things that might happen after certain types of acts; for example, if someone who cannot swim is thrown into a lake, then a likely consequence is that that person will get into difficulties and without help, might drown. The second point is that all of us, irrespective of our allegiance to a particular moral theory, need to take consequences into account, as Glover claims:

> Most of us, whether utilitarians or not, take some account of the likely effects of our actions on people's happiness, and we should all be in a mess if there was no correspondence between trying to make someone happier and succeeding.[8]

I need to stress here that I do not object to the term 'consequences' *per se*. Glover is correct in holding that, irrespective of our moral allegiance, one needs to take the consequences of acts into account. However, I do object to the excessive and restrictive over-focus on the notion of consequences that leads to the detriment of other morally important issues such as moral character and moral education. Furthermore, when people (e.g. nurses) have a superficial comprehension of 'consequences' and a crude understanding of the meaning and scope of consequentialism, not to mention its problems, then I find this state of affairs objectionable.

On the relationship between rightness and goodness, Frey believes that act-consequentialism is an example of a welfarist theory because

> rightness is made a function of goodness, and goodness is understood as referring to human welfare.[9]

This suggests that a good act is always a right act. For the moment, let us assume that this claim is true, there is still the question of how rightness is determined. In response to this question, Frey claims that act-consequentialism is

> impersonal and aggregative, in that rightness is determined by considering, impersonally, the increases and diminutions in well-being of all those affected by the act and summing those increases and diminutions across persons.[10]

At least three questions arise regarding the above that are far from simple to settle. First, how can one go about evaluating or measuring the various 'increases and diminutions in well-being'? 'Well-being'[11] is defined and conceived in different ways, including objective and subjective accounts, thus convergence is problematic. Some might argue that depending on which subjective account is provided, well-being cannot be measured. Second, is it possible to evaluate well-being for 'all those affected by the act'? This is clearly problematic; just how can one *know* which people have been or will be affected by each and every act? Third, act-consequentialism focuses on the impartial nature of morality; indeed impartiality is one of its central tenets. Act-consequentialism considers that the interests of strangers should count equally with those of one's loved ones, but here again problems arise, for example, what does it actually mean to treat someone impersonally and how can one go about this? This charge is commonly described as 'the nearest and dearest objection'. Taken together, these objections pose serious problems for act-consequentialism as a plausible moral theory.

In addition to act-consequentialism being a welfarist theory, Frey claims that act-consequentialism is also a maximizing theory:

> One concrete formulation of the principle of utility, framed in the light of welfarist considerations, is 'Always maximize net desire satisfactions.'[12]

Desire satisfactions[13] are interests that people desire as part of their lives. Examples include good health, relationships with others, pastimes and wealth. According to the above quote by Frey, one should maximize these interests on each and every occasion. But once again this is no simple matter, critics often pointing to the difficulty in always maximizing goods and benefits. As a way of avoiding such objections, some theorists have developed 'satisficing' versions of consequentialism, which claim that rather than aiming to *maximize* interests, people should aim to *satisfy* their interests. The moral requirement here is less stringent and these theorists argue that this version of consequentialism resolves one or more of the standard objections levelled at maximizing forms of consequentialism.

According to maximizing consequentialism, the goal is to maximize human welfare. This begs the question, how should one best go about achieving this? Since Hare's *Moral Thinking*,[14] it has been acknowledged that perhaps the best way of maximizing human welfare overall is to forego aiming to maximize it on each and every occasion. This view, however, contrasts sharply with utiltiarians such as J. Bentham and J. S. Mill. Bentham developed utilitarianism, an extreme form of consequentialism, as a political theory. Mill then adapted the theory. In its classical form, utilitarianism holds that maximizing utility for the majority of individuals is the *only* criterion for determining the morality of acts and omissions. It therefore places all of the moral emphasis upon the consequences of an act or omission. Mill states:

> The creed which accepts as the foundation of morals 'utility' or 'the greatest happiness principle' holds that acts are right in proportion as they tend to promote happiness; wrong as they tend to promote the reverse of happiness. By happiness is intended pleasure and the absence of pain; by unhappiness, pain and the privation of pleasure.[15]

Objections to act-consequentialism

Some brief critical comments regarding act-consequentialism have already been made. I shall now examine in more depth possible objections to act-consequentialism or act-utilitarianism.

The neglect of moral character

This criticism targets an omission of act-consequentialism and other obligation-based moral theories including deontology. I make this point early in this book because it is important to my claims in the remainder of the book. The notion of adequacy in relation to moral theories helps determine one's views and preferences about the plausibility of particular moral theories. For example, it partly explains why some thinkers prefer obligation-based moral theories to character-based ethics. Rachels believes that an adequate moral theory

> must provide an understanding of moral character; and second, that modern moral philosophy has failed to do this.[16]

I accept this claim without reservation; indeed this claim motivates much of this book. The reason why I believe moral theories must provide a satisfactory account of moral character is because I view ethics as a discipline that is primarily concerned with how people ought to respond to the interests of others and how people can get on in life. For example, do they fare well or badly? Without a plausible account of moral character – the kind of person one is, demonstrable by the cultivation and exercise of traits of character, both virtues and vices, and one's motives for action – this particular debate regarding morality, the virtues and human responsiveness will be stifled. I discuss moral character in relation to general ethics in more detail in Chapter 5 and in relation to nursing practice in Chapters 8 and 10.

Anti-theory and the assumption that moral dilemmas are resolvable

Act-consequentialism focuses, restrictively so, on the notions of 'right action' and 'morally right action' (this also applies to act-utilitarianism and deontology). According to these moral theories, 'ethics' is often conceived as a search for 'right' and 'wrong' answers to moral dilemmas. The aims of moral theory are not clear-cut; indeed there is disagreement on this in the literature. Sensible questions include: 'What should moral theories do?' and 'What do moral agents expect, want and need from moral theories?' Williams,[17] for example, believes that it is unrealistic to expect even hybrid moral theories to resolve moral dilemmas because the moral life is too richly textured and complex for this to be achievable. As noted, obligation-based moral theories at their core strive to provide action-guidance and develop some kind of decision procedure to help people settle or resolve moral dilemmas. Traditional versions of consequentialism and deontology fail to account for other aspects of the moral life that are clearly important. I believe that Williams is acknowledged by some others as an 'anti-theorist', which essentially means that he would reject the claim 'the pivotal aim and role of a moral theory is to provide people with action guidance'.

The neglect of moral remainder

Hursthouse, a virtue ethicist, would agree with Williams. Hursthouse has examined the large body of philosophical literature on moral dilemmas, including the possibility that there are, or could be, 'irresolvable' dilemmas. The latter are described as situations 'where doing x and doing y are *equally* [my italics] wrong, but one has to do x or y, or one in which two moral requirements conflict but neither overrides the other'.[18] Hursthouse also discusses another important yet neglected topic in ethics namely the subject of 'moral remainder'. The notion of moral remainder and its link with virtue ethics is an important thread running through this book. I will therefore spend a little time describing it. Hursthouse explains the idea of moral remainder thus:

> Suppose there are irresolvable dilemmas and someone is faced with one. Then, whatever they do, they violate a moral requirement, and we expect them (especially when we think in terms of real examples) to register this in some way – by feeling distress or regret or remorse or guilt, or, in some cases, by recognizing that some apology or restitution or compensation is called for.[19]

This emotional response – the remorse, guilt, distress or need for restitution – is the moral remainder, i.e., the moral agent's emotions during and after an irresolvable dilemma. Moreover, Hursthouse believes that dilemmas thought clearly *resolvable* are resolvable *only* with the moral remainder. This is because the moral requirement that is overridden retains considerable moral and emotional force. Besides the first body of literature on moral dilemmas, Hursthouse has also examined a second body of literature on dilemmas in applied ethics. She gives an example of this type of dilemma: Should the intensive care doctor lie to the patient who survived a car crash which killed the rest of her immediate family? Hursthouse believes that this second body of literature nearly always ignores the first. She holds that the contributors to this literature appear not to 'even entertain the possibility that the dilemma they are discussing is irresolvable'.[20] Indeed the assumption appears to be that there is one correct decision that the theorists' chosen moral theory – usually deontology or utilitarianism – will discover. Furthermore, Hursthouse believes that the contributors neglect to mention moral remainder, instead they focus almost exclusively on the question: 'Which is *the right* act in this case, *x* or *y*?'[21]

What accounts for this oversight in ignoring moral remainder in the applied ethics literature? Hursthouse believes that writers commit one of several fallacies and this helps to explain the terrible failure to discuss (or even mention) moral remainder. The first possible fallacy is 'the false dilemma'. This occurs when the writer 'take[s] the dilemma to be "*either x* is the morally right act to do here (without qualification) and *y* is the one that's morally wrong *or y* is the morally right act (without qualification), etc"'.[22] A third possibility is ignored, for example, 'Well, they are both pretty awful, but (supposing the dilemma is resolvable) *x* isn't quite as bad as *y*.'[23] Hursthouse claims that in moral dilemmas people assume there is one side that is unreservedly morally right and the other side is simply wrong. This assumption runs, as Hursthouse notes, deep in ordinary common sense morality and extends to conflicts between two different people. Hursthouse asks: 'Why is the fallacy harder to see when the choice is between two courses of action?'[24] Her response is that in part this concerns confusing 'two different senses of the phrases "morally right decision", or "right moral decision"'.[25] In the following quote, Hursthouse illustrates one way in which these phrases are used:

> Suppose we have a moral dilemma which is resolvable *x* is worse than *y*. Then the decision to do *y* rather than *x* is, in the circumstances, the *right* decision. Moreover (supposing the decision to have been made on the moral grounds that *x* is worse than *y*), it is a moral

decision, or one that has been made morally. So it is the 'morally right decision' or the 'right moral decision'.[26]

There is a second different way of using the phrases 'morally right decision' and 'right moral decision'. This concerns the use of these phrases to mean a good deed or a morally right act. In Hursthouse's words:

> As such, it is an act that merits praise rather than blame, an act that an agent can take pride in doing rather than feeling unhappy about, the sort of act that decent, virtuous people do and seek out occasions for doing ... Moreover, people can take pride in deciding to do such actions – they are the sorts of decision that decent virtuous people make – and are praised for thus deciding, whether or not the act comes off. Suppose it does not come off, well, that is a pity, but still, we say, they made the 'morally right decision', the 'right moral decision'; good for them.[27]

Hursthouse believes that the difference still might not be easy to see, it is therefore useful to consider the following claim that helps to bring the difference out. The claim is: 'When morally right decisions come off – when the agent succeeds in doing what she intended to do – we get morally right action.'[28] This applies to the second way of using 'morally right decision'. But, according to Hursthouse, 'if we are using "morally right decision" in the first way, we cannot say this truly, for it is obviously false'.[29] Hursthouse gives the following example to illustrate:

> The man who has induced two women to bear a child of his by promising marriage, can only marry one, but he may not be in an irresolvable dilemma; it may be worse to abandon A than B, and let us suppose he makes 'the morally right decision' and marries A, perforce breaking his promise to B and condemning her child to illegitimacy. He merits not praise, but blame, for having created the circumstances that made it necessary for him to abandon B; he should be feeling ashamed of himself, not proud, and so on.[30]

The above scenario came about because of the man's intentional actions and desires. However, Hursthouse still thinks that when the case involves a dilemma brought about through no fault of the agent, the act chosen – the one evil thought marginally less evil than the other – will

> still not be a morally right or good act, not one that leaves her with those 'circumstances [so] requisite to happiness', namely 'inward peace of mind, consciousness of integrity, [and] a satisfactory review

of [her] own conduct' as Hume so nicely puts it. On the contrary, it will, or should, leave her with some sort of remainder.[31]

As noted, the resolution of dilemmas in applied ethics literature fails to mention moral remainder. Hursthouse believes that frequently the writers prevaricate on 'morally right decision' and this leads to a false dilemma. She is uncertain whether this difference between the two senses of 'morally right decision' and 'right moral decision' is concealed on purpose or the writers are truly ignorant of it in the first place. The latter is doubtful. It is possible that the writers have not thought about the use of 'morally right decision' and 'right moral decision' in the same way that Hursthouse clearly has. At any rate, there is confusion between two very different questions, namely, 'Which is the morally right decision, to do x or to do y? and 'Which is the morally right action ... x or y?'[32] Hursthouse speculates: '*If* there are no irresolvable dilemmas, the first question does not pose a false dilemma, but even if every moral dilemma is resolvable, the second certainly does, for the correct answer may well be "Neither".'[33] For example, during an armed bank robbery a hostage collapses, clutching his chest. The armed robber has to decide whether to (a) carry on mercilessly or (b) get medical help and allow the doctor access. He decides to do (b). This decision is, on Hursthouse's view, morally right because the hostage is helped; to carry on regardless would have been a greater evil. But one cannot say that the robber's action is morally right because he was acting viciously – robbing a bank is not a good deed – and he should feel guilt and be blamed for creating the situation in the first place. Perhaps the hostage would not have collapsed if the robber had not carried out this vicious act in the first place.

Problems with utilitarianism

Ignoring other peoples' rights

The aforementioned quote by Mill (p. 44) makes it quite clear that utilitarianism – in all its forms – is no ally to the individual. This point has been picked up on by other moral theorists, especially rights-based theorists who argue that utilitarian thinking often leads to a violation or overriding of peoples' rights. For instance, because the interests of the many outweigh (or negate) the interests of the few, one's rights to autonomous decision-making can be violated or one's rights to freedom and liberty can be outweighed. An aspect of ordinary morality that requires some acknowledgement is that people very often do think according to crude utilitarianism or consequentialism. Imagine a disagreement where seven people claim that 'The Beatles' split up in 1969, while one person firmly believes it was 1970. The majority of individuals – the seven – would probably think they were correct and think that the other chap is wrong (of course, in this example the one chap would be correct). Or suppose a group of people are undecided which film to see at the cinema and it is agreed that the group shall not split up. Six out of ten want to see the new James Bond film, while the other four wish to see the latest film Noir by Hampton. This quandary might be resolved by the group of six people trotting off to see the Bond film, thus leaving four disgruntled film buffs (they had after all agreed to stay as a group). While these examples might appear trivial, they are representative of what occurs in our ordinary lives. I suppose some people would refer to this idea as 'strength in numbers', i.e., a viewpoint is somehow strengthened according to the number of people that make it. Certainly, people spend a considerable amount of time thinking about the consequences/outcomes of actions and perhaps a little less time thinking about the consequences/outcomes of omissions. This kind of thinking probably also includes some reflection on one's interests and the interests of others. What is quite clear is that the interests and rights of individuals could be ignored, violated or overridden by the conclusions of utilitarian reasoning.

No action-guidance until its second premise

Hursthouse has examined the first and second premises put forward by act utilitarianism and she has concluded that it is not until the second premise that one is given specific guidance on how to act morally, i.e., told what the right thing to do is. According to Hursthouse, a utilitarian might initially present her account of right action thus:

> P. 1. An action is right iff ['iff' means 'if and only if'; my words] it promotes the best consequences.[34]

However, despite the above premise that links the utilitarian concepts of 'right action' and 'best consequences', it fails to provide guidance on how to act. One must understand what counts as 'best consequences' for this to be so. Therefore a second premise, specifying this, must be provided. For example:

> P. 2. The best consequences are those in which happiness is maximized.[35]

The above premise forges the utilitarian link between 'best consequences' and 'happiness'. However, Hursthouse believes that the slogans used in utilitarianism do not succeed in singling out the most important notion because just as the 'Good' is singled out, so too (equally perhaps) could the concepts of 'happiness' or 'consequences'. Regarding the rather uninformative first premise of act-utilitarianism, Hursthouse thinks that this point is seldom, if ever, mentioned simply because people are so familiar with how utilitarians specify the notion of 'best consequences'. But while the second premise of utilitarianism routinely offers no surprises, according to Hursthouse it is possible that obscure things could emerge. For example:

> Someone might specify the 'best consequences' as those in which the number of Roman Catholics was maximized (and the number of non-Catholics minimized). Or someone might specify the 'best consequences' as those in which certain moral rules were adhered to.[36]

Hursthouse argues that it is this familiarity with utilitarianism and the ideas that people (intuitively) bring to the subject that help form and maintain this understanding of, for example, the meaning of 'best consequences'. The answer to 'What are best consequences?' is not given in the first premise of act-utilitarianism. But the gaps are filled in because each of us has a pretty good idea of what counts as 'a good consequence', namely something that will, for instance, produce pleasure or happiness or relieve suffering.

Utilitarianism's single rule and misrepresenting morality

Act-utilitarianism and other common conceptions of consequentialism provide just one rule: 'An act is right iff it maximizes best consequences.' A standard objection of utilitarianism is that in applying its single rule *without* the need for judgement, 'it misrepresents the texture of our moral experience, making it out to be much simpler than it really is'.[37] Hursthouse believes that because it fails to question whether or not its single rule does apply, fails to consider the plausibility of its extension and denies any higher order rules; it fails to

> capture the number of occasions where we want to say, 'This other (non-utilitarian) rule or consideration just *does* apply here, and it is not simply obvious that it is outranked by the rule about minimizing suffering, though I agree it sometimes is – don't you see?'[38]

Furthermore, as Hursthouse notes, the single rule of act-utilitarianism is couched in evaluative concepts such as 'happiness', 'well-being' and 'best consequences'. Utilitarians can resolve this problem by grounding their theory on empirical claims, for example, by defining 'happiness' as the satisfaction of preferences or desires. The single rule of utilitarianism is clearly evaluative; there are real problems for the utilitarian who makes, for instance, a distinction between the higher and lower pleasures.

There is another standard objection to utilitarianism as stated by Hursthouse: 'According to non-utilitarians, utilitarianism so frequently yields the wrong resolutions of hard cases.'[39] Hursthouse believes that it might be difficult to distinguish between the above two standard objections to utilitarianism. But she claims it is possible to see the difference. There are cases where deontologists (and virtue ethicists) agree with utilitarians that the right thing to do is to minimize suffering. But while the utilitarian simply thinks it adequate and sufficient to apply his single rule, deontologists (and virtue ethicists) think *getting* to this resolution is far from simple,

> for example, in order to avoid a great amount of suffering that would be brought about by keeping it, a promise had to be broken, is something that has to be taken into account; judgement has to be exercised to determine whether this was the sort of promise that could be broken and whether the good effects of doing so are sufficient to justify it, and so on.[40]

So according to this objection, deontologists (and virtue ethicists) claim it is wrong to equate the content and quality of our deliberations with the simple application of the utilitarians' single rule. This is a claim I fully endorse; indeed it is one of the prime motivations for this book.

Misrepresenting morality: Stocker[41] on modern moral theories' account of moral motivation

Stocker is dissatisfied with modern moral theories, including utilitarianism and deontology, for not providing a rich account of the moral life. According to Stocker, these theories *over* concentrate on actions and consequences. He is especially dismayed with obligation-based theories because they fail to examine moral motives. Or they provide an account of moral motivation – crudely, the motives for one's actions, thoughts and feelings – that is so wrapped up in inflexible and strict obligations that it provides an unsatisfactory account of moral motivation. The latter account can be described as 'unnatural' and 'unconvincing'.

A pivotal example from Stocker illustrates this point very well, thus I make no apologies for quoting at length:

> You are in a hospital, recovering from a long illness. You are very bored and restless and at loose ends when Smith comes in again. You are now convinced more than ever that he is a fine fellow and a real friend – taking so much time to cheer you up, travelling all the way across town, and so on. You are so effusive with your praise and thanks that he protests that he always tries to do what he thinks is his duty, what he thinks will be best. You at first think he is engaging in a polite form of self-deprecation, relieving the moral burden. But the more you two speak, the more clear it becomes that he was telling the literal truth; that it is not essentially because of you that he came to see you, not because you are friends, but because he thought it his duty, perhaps as a fellow Christian or Communist or whatever, or simply because he knows of no one more in need of cheering up and no one easier to cheer up.[42]

How would one feel if this happened? Would one be pleased to hear Smith's motive for his visit? Most probably, one would be disappointed and rather upset to hear that Smith did not visit because he wanted to be a good friend or because he really liked you and was concerned about your health. His act appears calculating. In relation to Smith's motive, Stocker says, 'surely there is something lacking here – and lacking in moral merit or value'.[43] Smith's actions appear good, even kind. But his motive is the problem. The motivation for his visit is an abstract sense of duty, 'to do the right thing'. People form friendships and relationships with others that are mutually valuable and beneficial; friendships ought to be made and maintained *for their own sakes* not because one perceives there is an obligation to do so. Would one wish to be like Smith? Would one wish Smith to be one's friend? Would one wish to live among people like Smith? The answer to these questions is surely in the negative and an emphatic one at that. And yet, theories of obligation such as consequentialism and deontology focus almost exclusively on the idea that people *must* obey certain moral obligations.

Act-consequentialism and the problem of intuitions

An important objection of act-consequentialism (and consequentialism in general) concerns the way it creates conflicts with or at least fails to accommodate some of our moral intuitions. We hold intuitions about a wide range of actions, beliefs and practices. Frey gives the following as examples:

> Frown upon murdering or torturing someone, upon enslaving people or using them as means, upon acting in certain contexts and so using people in certain ways for mere marginal increases in utility, all of which act-utilitarianism is supposed to (be able to) license.[44]

Although some intuitions are deeper, more sound than others, the above are all deep-rooted examples of moral intuitions found in Western liberal society. Critics of act-consequentialism, for example, deontologists and virtue ethicists, hold that other moral theories can better account for (at least) some of these intuitions. All of these intuitions appear to relate in some way to our respect for persons' lives. As this is a sound and fundamental moral notion, it is particularly interesting to ask: How does act-consequentialism license these intuitions concerning the rightness of acts? The answer lies with another of consequentialism's main tenets: the act-consequentialist is compelled to call acts right if they produce better actual consequences than other alternative acts. For example, if it is thought that act x – to murder a dictator who is responsible for the deaths of thousands of innocent people – will produce the best consequences among three options (x, y, z), then act x, because its consequences are better than y or z, would be the morally right act to perform. However, Frey responds to this form of reasoning by claiming that this conclusion 'conflicts with our moral intuitions or ordinary moral convictions'.[45]

Utilitarianism: Impartialism and conflicts between intuitions

I shall discuss the above ideas in a little more depth. People have a range of different interests and needs. However, despite this variety, utilitarianism insists that when deciding what to do, one ought to consider and rate everyone's interests as equally important. Mill believes that

> utilitarianism requires [the person] to be as strictly impartial as a benevolent and disinterested spectator.[46]

Mill has his supporters, for example, in the first chapter of *The Elements of Moral Philosophy*,[47] Rachels writes about impartiality and calls it a fundamental moral requirement. But why is the notion about impartiality so important in our moral lives? Why should John be impartial towards his wife, Helen? The basis of close relationships, family and marriage is love, affection and partiality between those involved. People tend to be partial towards their spouse, family, close friends and colleagues. Is there anything wrong with mothers who love their children, care for them, put them first and protect them above all else? Parents tend to care for their own children in ways that they do not care for other children. Parents behave partially towards their children all or nearly all of the time. What is wrong with this? Is this not an important characteristic of being a 'good' parent? If parents were not partial, their children might be ignored, feel neglected or even harmed in some way. The same thing applies to how each of us treats our friends. Partialism is a feature of friendship; it is expected between friends. For instance, Sam would rescue his best friend, Jake, but he might well pass by a stranger in need because Jake has not met this person and feels no affinity towards him. An important part of our moral lives concerns friendships with and affection for others. Moral theories such as utilitarianism that urge impartiality find it difficult to account for these aspects of the moral life. Indeed utilitarianism provides a crude, simplistic account of this aspect of the moral life, thus failing to portray real life as it is. Critics of act-consequentialism argue that there are many moral intuitions that support partiality towards loved ones and ourselves, i.e., that one should put one's own interests and those of loved ones ahead of others, especially strangers. This idea appears sensible since we are morally responsible for our own lives. But while one can help others including strangers and aid their distress, one is not morally responsible for the course of others' lives. And of course if one neglects one's own life, one might be unable or less able to help others. In sum, critics claim that act-consequentialism produces conflicts with or fails to accommodate some of our deeper moral intuitions.

But what about those occasions when moral intuitions and the claims made by consequentialism coincide? Frey believes this omission is noteworthy. One explanation why this might be so is that the critic of act-consequentialism somehow believes that these established intuitions are either compatible with or are produced from his theory of the right. Two possible positions emerge from this,

> on one of which rightness has nothing whatever to do with an act's consequences and on the other of which the rightness of certain acts has nothing whatever to do with an act's consequences.[48]

It will become clear in this book that virtue ethics is an example of the first position. Frey notes a third position that is not anti-consequentialist.

This view holds that the rightness of an act concerns its consequences plus something else, for example, the motive from which the act was performed. This view is a hybrid account of right action. While it might not be anti-consequentialist, its action-guidance will depend on the moral force given to the motives that are taken into account when determining the rightness or wrongness of the act.

Which intuitions are deeper than others?

It was noted earlier that some moral intuitions are thought more secure or deeper than others. Indeed, according to Frey, some philosophers believe that certain deeper intuitions are truer than any normative moral theory. This begs a couple of questions, one of which I will deal with and the other I will put to one side. First, I will set aside the question of whether moral intuitions have probative force in ethics.[49] I will instead deal with the following question: which intuitions are more secure than others and why? Although critical thinking is required here, according to Frey, irrespective of which critical methodology is adopted some intuitions survive intense critical scrutiny. Rawls[50] believes that if one's chosen moral theory produced a result that was contrary to one's deep intuitions, for example, if slavery was justified by the theory, then this provides sufficient reason for one to revise or amend the theory. Another problem arises in clarifying which moral intuitions are more secure or deeper than others, namely that there is disagreement because of factors such as cultural diversity and gender differences. Whatever the reason though, the outcome is that thinkers side with different intuitions concerning particular acts or classes of acts which they regard as crucial. Therefore the goal of arriving at just one or two deep and secure intuitions is complicated. Problems remain, in my view, regarding exactly how one can compare the deepness or correctness of moral intuitions. The fact that several 'crucial' intuitions are proposed, I believe, indicates wide variation and a lack of consensus among thinkers; and holding more than one or two reduces the strength of the intuitionist's claims. One also needs to note the effect of historical eras on one's willingness to label some intuitions as more favourable or correct than others. For example, Frey believes that whereas truth telling and promise keeping were once highly favourable secure intuitions to hold, nowadays opinion has altered somewhat. Nowadays, Frey claims that the wrongness of abortion has *perhaps* [my italics] taken over as one of the more secure contemporary moral intuitions. However, there is no empirical evidence for this; indeed Frey provides no reasons in support of his claim. However, he does believe that one's moral intuitions depend, to a large extent, upon one's political orientation:

> Someone who is politically conservative not uncommonly puts the wrongness of abortion into the favoured class, whereas political liberals are very unlikely to agree.[51]

Perhaps, then, Frey believes that the secure moral intuition regarding the wrongness of abortion is true *if* one is a conservative. Because of the large number of conservative voters, Frey might firmly believe that there are many people who would hold and defend this moral intuition. However, this discussion demonstrates the difficulty in defending moral claims, in this case concerning assumptions regarding the number of people holding a moral intuition about the wrongness of abortion. Whatever the disagreements between the scope, depth and limits of moral intuitions, attacks on act-consequentialism are very often launched because of the assumption that some intuitions remain despite critical scrutiny. It is hard to see how such intuitions as 'slavery is morally justifiable' could survive once rigorous critical examination has been conducted. Indeed, as discussed above, an intuition of this kind would probably require an amendment in the moral theory that grounds it. If an intuition survived critical reflection, it would most probably be a legitimate and defensible one. Motivated by this problem regarding intuitions, theorists have aimed to develop act-consequentialism by incorporating all manner of conceptual devices into the structure of the theory. The aim is that results can then be obtained in particular cases that are more compatible with the deep and secure intuitions identified by critics of act-consequentialism. According to Frey, Sidgwick is an example of the aforementioned kind of thinker. In Book IV of *The Methods of Ethics*,[52] Sidgwick aims to convince readers that act-consequentialism does indeed provide support for aspects of commonsense morality, although he admits that there are parts and details of the theory that are incompatible with commonsense morality and hence require reformulation. Sidgwick took the view that amending act-consequentialism was necessary to respond to some of the conflicts between the application of act-consequentialism and the views taken to be representative of commonsense morality. This view is in opposition to the hard line utilitarian view adopted by Smart.[53] However, according to Sidgwick, it remains the case that act-consequentialism is unable to sweep aside all of commonsense morality so that regarding justice, for example, act-consequentialism should give way.

Intuitions – The need for supporting argumentation

This debate over the correctness of moral intuitions leaves me wondering how two claims can be squared. On the one hand, Rawls claims that slavery is morally unjustifiable and that nothing more needs to be said to defend this position. And on the other hand, the idea that moral philosophy, or more strictly philosophical analysis, is intended to be a rigorous pursuit that aims to search for and defend secure foundations for moral beliefs. One is left with the feeling that Rawls has not been successful here, or at least he fails to go far enough, basically further justification is required here concerning the legitimacy and justification of his claim regarding slavery. This would be true even if one agrees (as I do) with his view that slavery is morally wrong. Supporting reasons need to be given for one's beliefs to allow others to critically evaluate them. It is possible that one could hold deep moral intuitions that others might abhor, for example, extreme racist views. It is therefore crucial that supporting argumentation is provided that allows for critical scrutiny and probing examination. If commonsense morality with its secure moral intuitions about particular acts is a plausible view, then this provides problems for act-consequentialism. Despite epistemological concerns, for example, concerning the justification of moral intuitions, I accept that people often hold deep intuitions about a range of acts in the world including the wrongness of murder, slavery and torture. Act-consequentialists are motivated to bring their theory into line with some of these deeper moral intuitions. However, as a result of doing so, act-consequentialists minimize their theory's merits, for example, its alleged simplicity. (However, it is arguable whether consequentialism, especially the utilitarianism of Smart, could be accurately described as a 'simple' moral theory.) Nevertheless, viewing act-consequentialism as a plausible moral theory would be further hampered if it failed to account for some deeper moral intuitions, especially those thought too secure to be mistaken.

Merits of consequentialism

It avoids the charge of moral relativism

Proponents of act-utilitarianism allege that one of its merits is that it avoids the charge of moral relativism that affects deontology (and as we shall see, virtue ethics). This is because act-utilitarianism's first premise (unlike deontology's) contains just one rule: 'An action is right if it produces the best consequences.' One then needs to know what 'best consequences' means. This information is given in its second premise 'best consequences are those that maximize happiness'; therefore it is plausible to suggest that act-utilitarianism is not guilty of moral relativism.

Consequentialism is codifiable

Another feature of consequentialism (and deontology) is that they aim to be codifiable, i.e., these theories hold that ethics should be conceived as a set of moral obligations, rules and principles that provide specific action-guidance. This is held, almost assumed, to be one of consequentialism's merits. Pincoffs[54] notes that this was the dominant view of a normative ethics. According to Hursthouse, codifiability means that universal obligations, rules and principles possess two features:

> (a) they would amount to a decision procedure for determining what the right action was in any particular case; (b) they would be stated in such terms that any non-virtuous person could understand and apply then correctly.[55]

Hursthouse calls this 'the strong codifiability thesis' (SCT). While this feature can be seen in a positive light, one can also understand that it could, if other morally important features were forgotten, prove objectionable.

Rule-consequentialism

Rule consequentialism has arisen and developed in no small part because of the flaws in act-consequentialism regarding its conflicts with some secure moral intuitions. Rule-consequentialism develops rules that are judged morally right if the consequences of adopting such rules are thought more favourable than unfavourable to the majority of people. Rule consequentialism does not judge or test the morality of particular actions, rather it tests the morality of rules such as 'lying is wrong' or 'stealing is wrong'. Adopting rules such as these is usually thought favourable for everyone. Because it does not target specific acts, rule consequentialism provides more general action-guidance for people compared to the single rule of act-consequentialism. However, does rule-consequentialism fare better than act-consequentialism? Not according to Frey, who believes that in at least the versions of rule-consequentialism known to him, it 'has long been known to suffer from certain types of instabilities that seem irreducibly part of the theory'.[56] This view is shared by Lyons[57] who claims that rule-consequentialism collapses into act-consequentialism. It is certainly true that in avoiding the problems associated with act consequentialism, new problems are created for rule consequentialism. For example, under rule consequentialism it might be thought socially beneficial to introduce a rule prohibiting slavery. However, it is possible that 'on balance, a rule permitting slavery actually produces more benefit for society'.[58] Part of the problem is that once one agrees that certain moral intuitions have an important role to play in morality and once one thinks that some of these intuitions are true, it becomes more difficult to accommodate these intuitions within a consequentialist structure. In other words, rather than trying to maintain some sort of consequentialist theory, it might be more profitable to turn to moral intuitionism instead. Given this and the importance of deeper moral intuitions, it might be that a non-consequentialist moral theory could better accommodate these intuitions. Critics of both kinds of consequentialism (and more specifically, act and rule utilitarianism) suggest that this flaw – consequentialism's inability to accommodate deeper moral intuitions – explains why these forms of moral theory have failed to catch on. I accept that the conflict produced by act-consequentialism with regard to some deeper moral intuitions is a serious problem. But I would disagree with the assertion that act-consequentialism has not caught on. Of course, a lot depends on precisely what is meant by 'to catch on'. But from electronic searches of the general ethics literature, it is evident that obligation-based moral theories in general and consequentialism in particular are popular, if not to say dominant, theories. (The nursing literature searches produced very similar results – this will be discussed in Chapter 7.)

Consequentialism – Conclusions

Consequentialism clearly demarcates between right and wrong acts. It provides, at least on some accounts, a simple and intuitively appealing explanation of what makes right acts right and wrong acts wrong. However, consequentialism has been criticized on the grounds that it can be difficult for people to foresee *all* of the possible consequences of *all* of one's acts/omissions; indeed, it is hard to know what the consequences of acts/omissions will be even in reasonably straightforward cases. Act-consequentialists have responded to these (and other) criticisms with several strategies that go some way to accommodating deeper moral intuitions. However, the versions of consequentialism that I have discussed have three things in common. First, they aim to provide action-guidance. Second, they aim to develop decision procedures. And, third they aim to provide an account of the Right. In my view, however, more damaging is the fact that these theories either completely ignore or minimize the importance of several other morally important features including moral character, moral education and the role of the emotions in the moral lives of persons. I have noted several objections are commonly levelled at the *content* of consequentialist theories. Furthermore, because of these serious *omissions* I argue that act and rule consequentialism are incomplete and thus inadequate moral theories.

Deontology[59]

Deontological theories can be characterized as 'backward looking'. These theories again begin with: 'Act x is right if ____', but instead of filling in the blank with reference to the consequences of an act, they typically claim that what makes right acts right (and wrong acts wrong) are other morally important features that occur at the same time as or before the act. However, as with consequentialists who often disagree over what the good and bad consequences are, or who the recipients of the consequences should be or whether such a theory should be a maximizing theory, deontologists often disagree over what these morally important features are. For example, some insist that moral principles that encapsulate the intention or motive behind the act should be paramount, others look to divine commands and yet others look to intuitions. Agreement however is reached on one idea: 'The end doesn't always justify the means.' In other words, good consequences alone are not sufficient to make an act morally right and conversely, bad consequences do not necessarily make an act morally wrong.

Contemporary deontology[60]

To promote an understanding of deontology, it is fruitful to look closely at differences between deontological and consequentialist moral theories. It is clear from the above introduction that deontologists believe that there are some acts that are intrinsically wrong; wrong because of the sort of act they are. These sorts of acts are, irrespective of the consequences, morally unacceptable and impermissible. Even ends that might appear morally admirable cannot legitimately be achieved by these unacceptable means. According to Davis, deontologists hold that

> acting morally, or as we ought to act, involves the self-conscious acceptance of some (quite specific) constraints or rules that place limits both on the pursuit of our own interests and of our pursuit of the general good.[61]

Deontologists tend to agree that it is not morally required for persons to (a) always aim to promote their own interests or (b) pursue the general good. Deontologists think morality is largely a matter of sufficiency and neither of these two pursuits provides sufficient moral grounds for action. Deontologists are dissatisfied with consequentialism for several reasons, most of which have been noted in the previous section. Furthermore, according to deontologists, consequentialist theories can be criticized on the grounds that they encourage or allow us to sometimes treat other humans in inhumane ways. Deontologists often allege that such consequentialist theories misunderstand or misinterpret what it is to be a person.

Rawls argues that theories of right action can be exhausted by reference to just two categories: teleological and deontological. He writes:

> The two main concepts of ethics are those of the right and the good ... The structure of a moral theory is, then, largely determined by how it defines and connects these two basic notions ... The simplest way of relating them is taken by teleological theories: the good is defined independently from the right, and the right is defined as that which maximizes the good.[62]

Rawls contrasts a deontological theory with a teleological theory in two ways. First, the former do not 'specify the good independently from the right'[63] and second, deontological theories do not 'interpret the right as maximizing the good'.[64] Fried goes further on the relationship between the good and the right:

> The goodness of the ultimate consequences does not guarantee the rightness of the acts which produced them. The two realms are not only distinct for the deontologist, but the right is prior to the good.[65]

At least three things can now be said about deontologists' views on the right and the good. First, the Right is not definable in terms of the Good. Second, the claim 'the Good is prior to the Right' is rejected. And third, there is no necessary link between doing right and doing good.

For deontologists, acting right is concerned with refraining from doing things that are known (before the fact) to be wrong. Davis refers to these as 'deontological constraints', i.e., requirements that restrain us from doing certain acts. These include various laws, rules, principles, prohibitions, proscriptions and limitations. According to deontology, persons are obliged to refrain from doing acts known to be wrong

> even when they foresee that their refusal to do such things will clearly result in greater harm (or less good).[66]

Two obvious observations can now be made: first, deontological views are non-consequentialist and second, the former are non-comparative and non-maximizing. According to a deontologist, the wrongness of telling lies has nothing to do with the possible bad consequences of telling a particular lie or the general negative effects of lying. Rather, the wrongness of telling lies on the deontological view is

> because of the sorts of things they are, and are thus wrong even when they foreseeably produce good consequences.[67]

As noted, consequentialist theories are based on an impartial consideration of others' interests or welfare, while deontological views clearly are not. Davis provides an example that clarifies this point: imagine a scenario whereby one might harm one innocent person to prevent the deaths of five innocent people. If a deontologist refuses to harm the one, knowing fully well that this (impermissible) act would prevent five innocent deaths, then this clearly shows that the interests of the six do not count or at least do not count equally. If this is the case, i.e., their interests were all taken into account equally, then this act (to harm the one) would not only be permissible, but most probably obligatory. However, peoples' interests are complex and cannot be satisfactorily perceived and evaluated in this crude way. This point is noted by deontology; deontological views are not based on an impartial consideration of interests. As Davis explains:

> For that [impartially considering interests] would seem to allow – if not require – that each one of the five's interests be weighed against those of the one; it would seem to allow – if not require – us to (for example) toss a coin five times, in order for each of the five's interests to receive the same consideration that the one's interests are accorded.[68]

There is another area in which deontological views differ from consequentialist impartiality. Deontologists insist that one is not allowed to violate a deontological constraint by doing a particular act

> even when our doing so would obviate the necessity of five other people being faced with the decision to violate a deontological constraint or allow even more serious harm to occur.[69]

Deontologists hold that it is forbidden to harm one innocent person to decrease the number of deaths. Moreover it is forbidden to harm one person to decrease the number of killings carried out by other people who possess the moral character and motivations considered no worse than ours. As noted earlier, consequentialists hold that everyone's interests including one's own should be judged impartially. Thus one could claim that the stringent tenet of impartialism leads consequentialism to deprive or minimize one of personal autonomy. A consequentialist assesses his own interests, in effect, his life, as no more important than the interests of a total stranger. But Davis claims that if one is to have and sustain a life worth living, one ought to assign more weight to one's own interests simply because one's interests form one's life.[70] This favouritism is more than just tolerated by deontologists, for example, respecting personal autonomy may mean that one prioritizes and gives more weight to one's own interests and concerns compared to those of others. Deontological views provide more weight to one's own avoidance of wrongdoing ('wrongdoing' here means a violation of deontological constraints), compared to the interests and lives of others. Moreover, deontological views

> require that we assign more weight to our own avoidance of wrongdoing than we do to the avoidance of wrongdoing *tout court*, or the prevention of wrongdoing to others.[71]

Ultimately by a deontologist's lights, the preservation of one's moral integrity and excellence is not only more important than the preservation of others' lives, it is also more important than the preservation of others' moral integrity and excellence. Commenting on this issue, Davis remarks:

> We may not save a life with a lie even when the lie would prevent the loss of life by deceiving an evil agent who credibly intends to kill several innocent victims.[72]

Deontological constraints

There are three features of deontological constraints – the system of prohibitions and rules that form the basis of deontological views – that require closer inspection. These constraints are (a) usually formed as negative formulations, (b) usually narrowly framed and bounded and (c) usually narrowly directed. Each of these will now be discussed in a little more detail.

Deontological constraints – negative formulations

Deontological constraints are usually formulated as 'Thou shalt nots' or prohibitions. While it might be theoretically possible to transform these negative prohibitions into positive prescriptions – for example, 'do not tell lies' would become 'tell the truth' – deontologists regard the latter as inequivalent to negative prohibitions. While the deontologist is aware that the same bad or untoward consequences might arise from 'lying' and 'failing to tell the truth' and that these kinds of acts might arise from the same kind of motivations, it is also clear that 'lying' and 'failing to tell the truth' are not the same kinds of act (another example would be 'harming' and 'failing to benefit'). 'Kinds of acts' are the objects which deontologists deem right or wrong. It will therefore be possible for a deontologist to forbid 'lying' (one kind of act), while perhaps being ambivalent on 'failing to tell the truth' (a closely related but different kind of act). On this Fried thinks:

> In every case the [deontological] norm has boundaries and what lies outside those boundaries is not forbidden at all. Thus lying is wrong, while withholding a truth which another needs may be perfectly permissible – but that is because withholding a truth is not lying.[73]

Deontological constraints – Narrowly framed and bounded

The second feature of note is that deontological constraints are usually narrowly framed and bounded. This means that a person's obligations and other deontological views are explained in narrow terms and quite restrictive. Davis believes that this is important because one's understanding of a person's obligations and responsibilities will depend, in part, upon one's understanding of the scope of deontological constraints. And, as she notes, this will include various potentially contrasting views on what constitutes different kinds of acts.

Deontological constraints – Narrowly directed

The third feature of note is that deontological constraints are narrowly directed. This means that these constraints attach narrowly or specifically to peoples' decisions and acts, rather than generally to any of the possible consequences of their decisions and acts.[74] On this point, Nagel says: 'Deontological reasons have their full force against your doing something – not just against its happening.'[75]

Intention and foresight in deontology

The distinction between intention and foresight is often used to help explain the narrow-directedness of deontological constraints. This distinction holds that only if one intentionally harms another does one violate the constraint against harming the innocent. If for some reason, one chooses not to take action to prevent harm befalling others, then this is not a violation of the deontological constraint against harming the innocent. This remains the case if the harm that befalls someone is foreseen as a possible consequence of one's permissible action, as long as one's action was not a chosen means or towards a chosen end. However, one's action might be open to criticism on other grounds. According to deontological views and expressed in commonsense morality:

> We are not as responsible for (or not fully agent of) the foreseen consequences of our acts, as we are for the things we intend.[76]

As noted earlier, the majority of deontology's obligations are formulated negatively as prohibitions or impermissibles. For deontologists, the category of the impermissible is fundamental because it grounds the definition of the obligatory: 'What is obligatory is what it is impermissible to omit.'[77] However, it is unclear what people are obliged to do. Nevertheless, agreement surrounds the idea that people need to devote most of their time and energy to the realm of the permissible. On this, Fried remarks:

> One cannot live one's life by the demands of the domain of the right. After having avoided wrong and doing one's duty, an infinity of choices is left to be made.[78]

A stark contrast emerges between consequentialism and deontology. For consequentialists, the notion of the Right is strong and prior to the Good, while for deontologists the Right is usually held to be a weaker notion; deontologists tend to make the Good prior to the Right. As we have seen, in general terms consequentialism holds that a course of action is permissible

> when and only when it is the best (or equal best) option open to an agent: it is never permissible to do less good (or prevent less harm) than one can.[79]

Thus in a sense, consequentialists achieve what Davis calls moral closure: 'Every course of action is either right or wrong (and actions are permissible only if they are right)';[80] this 'simplicity' is seen as one of the merits of consequentialism. Contrast this with deontology's views: an act might be permissible without it being the best act or even a good option. The aforementioned tenet of consequentialism attracts criticism because it ensures that consequentialism is a strenuous and rigid moral theory; there is a lack of what Davis calls 'moral breathing room'. In short, according to deontologists consequentialism makes mistakes concerning the notions of permission, obligation and the Right.

Deontology and the doctrine of double effect

Although there are problems surrounding the tenability of the distinction between intention and foresight, many deontologists appeal to this to provide a plausible meaning of narrow-directedness. In describing the 'doctrine of double effect', Nagel states:

> To violate deontological constraints one must maltreat someone else intentionally. The maltreatment must be something that one does or chooses, either as an end or as a means, rather than something one's acts merely cause or fail to prevent but that one doesn't aim at.[81]

If one did not intend to do the act in question, then one cannot legitimately be accused of violating a deontological constraint. One might have done something wrong, but if it was not one's chosen end or means then according to this doctrine, one has not done anything wrong at all. It is possible to see the connection between narrow-directedness and narrow framing. The prohibitory force of deontological constraints attaches only to those things intended. Given this, it is clear that, for example, a lie is a different kind of act than is a failure to tell the truth. Lies (as attempted deceptions) are necessarily intended, while failures to disclose the truth do not necessarily aim at deception. Furthermore, accept that the concept of intention is developed and explained in terms of choice as a means to an end. For example, something counts as an intentional harming of the innocent only if it – the harm – was chosen either as an end or a means to an end. If this plausible claim is accepted, then foreseen harms are different from harms chosen as a means to prevent others' harms. In Davis's words:

> If an agent harms one person in order to prevent five others from being killed in a rockslide, what he or she does is an intentional

harming, and thus violates a deontological constraint. But if the agent refuses to kill the one to save the five, then, since the deaths of the five are not the agent's chosen means or the agent's chosen end, there is no violation of a deontological constraint.[82]

Consequentialism faces problems because of its need to predict the consequences of an act. Does deontology avoid such practical problems? There is no need by deontology's lights to speculate about the possible consequences of an act since we know that deontologists believe that acts are wrong (or right) because of the sorts of acts they are. Possible lists of wrong acts drawn up by deontologists will have in common that in some way they violate one or more of the deontological constraints. Nagel provides perhaps a representative list:

> Common moral intuition recognizes several types of deontological reasons – limits on what one may do to people or how one may treat them. There are special obligations created by promises and agreements; the restrictions against lying and betrayal; the prohibitions against violating various individual rights, rights not to be killed, injured, imprisoned, threatened, tortured, coerced, robbed; the restrictions against imposing certain sacrifices on someone simply as a means to an end; and perhaps the special claim of immediacy, which makes distress at a distance no different from distress in the same room. There may also be a deontological requirement of fairness, of even-handedness or equality in one's treatment of people.[83]

While it might appear that deontologists fare better than consequentialists in this area of morality, some theoretical problems remain. If deontologists reject the link between an act being wrong (or right) and its bad (or good) consequences, then what is it about a wrong (or right) act that makes it wrong (or right)? In other words, why are the items on Nagel's list above, there? (And Nagel's list is fairly representative of deontology.) In reply, deontologists can appeal to several sources. For example, some deontologists appeal to common moral intuitions, while others appeal to religion, for instance, Judaeo–Christian teachings. However, deontological constraints are also derived from another more fundamental principle. This principle is frequently presented as something like 'it is morally obligatory to respect every person as a rational agent'. The foundation for this principle is held to lie in Kant's ethics although there is some blurring among interpretations. Donagan's formulation more closely follows deontology's format: 'It is impermissible not to respect every human being, oneself or any other, as a rational creature.'[84] According to many deontologists including Fried and Donagan, part of respecting others as rational creatures is that one should refrain from subjecting them to the sorts of treatment proscribed by deontological constraints; indeed this is framed as a moral requirement. Nagel goes further on this point. In his view, if one identifies certain sorts of conduct as evil – for example, harming a child so that her frightened babysitter reveals some piece of important, perhaps life-saving, information – then it is clear that this conduct is something that one must not do. According to Nagel, 'evil' conduct means that one should be moved to eliminate it rather than maintain it. He believes that if consequentialists allow that it is right to lie to or harm the innocent, then they have an unsatisfactory understanding of what evil means or what it is for someone to be evil. Furthermore, this is true even if one's desire and intention is to prevent greater harm or promote the greater good. Davis claims that none of the aforementioned sources – moral intuitions, religion or the principle of respect for persons – satisfactorily grounds deontological moral judgements; likewise Hursthouse believes that 'intuition' and 'perception' are 'entirely unsatisfactory notions'.[85] For example, take appeals to common morality. The picture of the universe, once thought true by the Church Fathers, is now widely rejected. It is now widely thought that the views of priests and monks that dominated early religious morality are punitive or prejudiced. Therefore, as Davis warns:

> If traditional common morality can easily be seen to have such weak parts, it is wise to be sceptical, or at least cautious, about other parts, and about the foundation that holds all the parts together.[86]

Problems with deontology

No action-guidance until its second premise

Hursthouse has examined the first and second premise of simple deontology (the kind of deontology known to many people, loaded with moral rules). She argues that as in act-consequentialism, it is not until the second premise of deontology that people are given specific action-guidance. In the second premise, one is given information on what counts as a correct moral principle, rule or duty (these three notions forge the link with right action in the first premise). As Hursthouse explains, there are several possible ways in which to describe a correct moral rule or principle, for example, it is one that 'is laid down on us by God' ... 'is universalizable' ... [or] 'would be the object of choice of all rational beings'.[87] Deontologists will defend and justify the specific rules that they believe are correct, for example, they might defend rules permitting or prohibiting euthanasia, coercion or suicide. But what does this turn on? The answer to this is not forthcoming. Moreover, Hursthouse believes that it is untrue to say that many versions of deontology '"begin with" the Right, for they [as noted above] use the concept of moral rule or principle to specify right action'.[88] She notes that Frankena discusses versions of what he calls 'extreme act-deontology' wherein a right action 'just *is* right'.[89]

Hursthouse believes that in deontology (as in consequentialism) one is so familiar with the moral obligations, rules or principles proposed. This familiarity grounds one's understanding of the content of the obligations, rules and principles given in the second premise of deontology. Furthermore, Hursthouse claims that one has a good idea what a correct moral principle or rule is; for, when this premise is given, we have in mind, for instance, 'Do not kill', 'Do not break promises' and 'Tell the truth.' But Hursthouse thinks one would be surprised to find contenders such as 'Purify the Arian race', 'Keep women in their proper place, subordinate to men', 'Kill the infidel.'[90] She points out, however, that each of these has at some point in time all unfortunately counted as 'correct' moral rules. In sum then, given the first premise of simple deontology one is not actually told what counts as a correct moral obligation, rule or principle. This gap in our understanding is filled in through our familiarity with what we believe a correct moral obligation etc. is.

Wrongful harming or the permissible causing of harm?

People have views about what sorts of acts are right and wrong, and beliefs regarding the limits and bounds of peoples' moral responsibilities for their deeds. These help us to determine whether an act that causes harm is viewed as a case of wrongful harming or merely the permissible causing of harm. Peoples' different normative moral views – about what one should do and how one should live – lead them to have different beliefs about this distinction. Thus, one who is swayed by consequentialism

> will see a refusal to lie to one person in order to prevent serious harm from befalling five other people as a case of wrongfully harming the five, while someone with less consequentialist leanings might not.[91]

Either way, when individuals try to follow deontological views – for example, 'avoid wrongful harming' – they will interpret these views differently and as a result, probably end up acting in different ways in their attempts to follow such guidelines.

Appealing to the notion of respect

It is also prudent to be cautious about appealing to a fundamental moral principle such as 'respect for persons'. The notion of respect commonly employed is far from transparent; indeed it appears that the conception of 'respect' or 'respect for rational persons' is used in a narrow, technical or legal sense. Moreover, this idea is not clarified when one talks about respecting persons as rational creatures. A lack of clarity also surrounds another feature of respect. According to deontological views, the requirement of respect is thought not to include 'respect for other beings as possessors of welfare'.[92] The reason for this omission is unclear. Remember that, according to deontological theories, one ought to allow five people to be killed by a rockslide rather than harm one person ourselves. But surely this entails serious disrespect for the lives of the five? It is hard to defend the technical, narrow account usually given to respect. Even if plausible defences of this account could be provided, Davis thinks another important question remains, 'Why should respect be seen as something that morally outweighs the requirement to further others' well-being?'[93] In other words, why does the obligation of beneficence usually rank lower than respect for other people? Consequentialists frequently come under attack for maintaining that 'as long as human beings can remain alive, the lesser of two evils is always to be chosen'.[94] In their defence, consequentialists claim that minimum conditions must be met for a life worthy of a human and these conditions cannot be sacrificed. While this consequentialist position is open to criticism, it is quite clear that deontologists fare little better. The deontological position maintains, for example, that the whole community should die rather than violate the deontological constraint 'refrain from killing the innocent'. Davis suggests that deontologists need to reflect on the reasoning behind the following scenario,

> a proposed effort to save hundreds of lives by (for example) killing one innocent person that constitutes a failure of respect so great that it is worth sacrificing all of those lives.[95]

The reasoning behind the above scenario appears to make little sense; at least it counters deep moral convictions relating to the moral responsibility for saving lives and generally promoting others' interests.

Criticisms of the doctrine of double effect and the distinction between intended and foreseen harm

Criticisms have been levelled at the principle of double effect and questions raised over the tenability of the distinction between intended and foreseen harm. These criticisms possess some merit and as such, create problems for contemporary deontology. In response, deontologists will either need to expand the scope of their prohibitions or they will need to admit that these prohibitions do not carry absolute or categorical force. However, if the first point is addressed then serious problems relating to conflicts between duties arise. And if the second point is tackled, then the very structure of deontological views is threatened. This is because if deontological constraints do not produce absolute or categorical force, then what sort of force do they possess? How would a person tell between an act that is forbidden and one that is not? When the absolute force is removed from deontological constraints, deontological views collapse into a type of moral pluralism or even worse, an intuitionist type of moral pluralism. However, according to Fried, deontologists do not believe it is justifiable to refuse to violate a deontological constraint when the consequences of such a refusal would be dire. On such extreme cases, Fried says:

> And so the catastrophic may cause the absoluteness of right and wrong to yield, but even then it would be a non sequitur to argue (as consequentialists are fond of doing) that this proves that judgements of right and wrong are always a matter of degree, depending on the relative goods to be attained and harms to be avoided. I believe, on the contrary, that the concept of the catastrophic is a distinct concept just because it identifies the extreme situations in which the usual categories of judgment (including the categories of right and wrong) no longer apply.[96]

But while allowing the violation of deontological constraints in extreme circumstances helps to prevent deontology from fanaticism, it also undermines it as a plausible moral theory. Adding a so-called catastrophe clause is particularly problematic. How does one goes about distinguishing a 'catastrophic' situation, one in which right and wrong no longer apply, from other situations that are 'only' deemed 'dreadful' where right and wrong do apply? I share Davis's concern with this arbitrary decision. Whether there are extreme circumstances or not, these decisions remain moral decisions. According to Davis, terrible circumstances do not relieve us of our obligation to act morally; indeed one could suggest that terrible situations place greater demands on people. But whether this is framed in terms of obligations, rules or principles or the exercise of virtues is quite another matter. The idea that the notions of right and wrong are somehow not applicable in dire circumstances is one that Davis believes 'encourages complacency ... It is one that any reasonable person ought to reject'.[97] I concur with her view. But from Chapter 5 onwards I suggest that one can also view morality in terms of acting well, i.e., exercising the virtues of, for example, kindness patience and justice. Or conversely, one can act badly, i.e., exercise the vices of, for example, cruelty, impatience and injustice.

Criticisms of deontology's rules

Hursthouse criticizes the rules of simple deontology. She makes three points. First, as we have seen the rules of consequentialism are partly based on evaluative concepts such as 'happiness'. The rules of deontology, for example on lying, are also evaluative and as such limit their ability to provide adequate action-guidance. Deontologists might try to claim that their rules are somehow empirical or non-evaluative, but Hursthouse[98] believes this would be a mistake. This is because most deontologists are keen to invoke principles of beneficence and non-maleficence. And as Hursthouse claims, these moral principles also rest on fairly evaluative concepts such as 'promote the *interests* of clients' and 'do no *harm* to clients'. Her second point concerns the exercise of judgement. She claims that adult deontologists need to think very hard about what constitutes 'promoting their well-being', 'respecting their autonomy' and 'harming someone' not because of their evaluative nature, but in relation to the need to exercise judgement. Hursthouse's third point concerns the so-called mother's-knee rules. These rules including 'Don't lie' and 'Keep promises' are only easy to apply when the cases are easy to resolve; once the cases become hard, so too does the understanding and application of the rules. Once again judgement is involved as is 'a grasp of such things as "the sort of promise that may be broken, or need not be kept, or (even) should not be kept and should never have been made"'.[99]

Deontology: A critique of rights

I shall now briefly critique the notions of rights.[100,101] Like many other notions in ethics – for example, the notion of 'best interests' – the notion of rights is often portrayed as simple, yet is complex. The notion of rights is a relatively recent idea. It is thought that rights emerged during the Enlightenment, crudely the period of history between the 16th and 18th centuries. Moral rights were conceived as a means of providing and protecting certain important liberties such as rights to freedom and preservation of life. Nowadays, both moral and legal rights are widespread especially in contemporary health care. The latter, for example, patients' rights to refuse treatment are grounded in common law. But moral rights such as 'the right to be respected as a rational person' are grounded in moral values and beliefs, which are clearly evaluative and subjective phenomena. Numerous moral and legal rights compete against each other. Thus conflicts between rights arise; these conflicts can be between two or more moral rights as well as moral and legal rights. However, it is not clear how to resolve these conflicts; indeed, it is not clear how one can *know* which rights one has and in what circumstances these rights can be overridden.

I have five main concerns with the notion of rights, which I shall now describe. First, in ethics one is concerned with moral, not legal rights and this fact is often overlooked. As noted, legal rights are encapsulated in common or statute law. Moral rights are not synonymous with legal rights. This fact needs recognition. Second, the origin and intended purpose of moral rights requires deeper scrutiny. For example, where do rights come from? Are they entitlements to certain things (for example, health care), liberties (for example, freedom) or generally claims for protection?[102] Third, I suggest that when rights are invoked, for example, in terms of justice, one needs to bear in mind one's corresponding moral responsibilities. For instance, if one has a moral right to have a coronary artery bypass operation, then one has a moral responsibility to ensure that both pre- and post-operatively one does everything possible to make the surgery successful. This might include stopping smoking before the operation. These corresponding moral responsibilities are fraught with tensions and are often neglected in discussions about rights. Fourth, another aspect of rights that causes me concern is the seemingly endless lists that are nowadays produced from people who want certain protections or feel entitled to *x* or *y*. For example, 'I surely have a right to smoke a cigarette in public' or 'I have a right to park my car in this space even though it's for a disabled person.' These are examples where one's corresponding responsibilities have been disregarded. Possessing rights should mean that one behaves *decently*, meaning that the interests and needs of other people should be taken into account. To close this section, I believe it is not so much the moral right in question that is problematic (as long as the right can be adequately justified, however, this is not always achieved), rather it is the manner in which people exercise 'their' rights that I find objectionable. Simply put, from a virtue ethics perspective moral rights can be exercised either virtuously (for instance, kindly) or viciously (for instance, cruelly). How we respond to other peoples' *requests* or *demands* for their perceived moral rights is of fundamental importance in morality. It seems to me that if one exercises her rights virtuously (for example, kindly or justly), this serves as an illustration of that person acting morally well. In terms of the protection of one's rights, the virtues of justice and respectfulness should help to ensure that justifiable moral and legal rights are not overridden without good reason.

Deontology and intuitions: A response

Before I conclude this chapter, I shall discuss a possible response from deontologists with regard to their dependence upon intuition to see whether they can overcome this problem. This dependence upon intuition is denied, at least by some deontologists, in an attempt to respond to this standard objection. These deontologists advocate the SCT noted earlier by Hursthouse. In her words:

> They suppose (a) that they have (or will be able to formulate in time) a complete and consistent set of rules in which second-order ranking rules or principles settle any conflicts among first-order rules, which have been formed with much more precision than the 'mother's-knee' versions, and which may also be supposed to have had many necessary exception clauses built into them. Such a system would determine what was required in every situation and (b) would not rely on intuition or insight to resolve conflicts.[103]

If the above albeit extravagant strategy is accepted, then it would appear that deontology could solve the conflict problem without dependence upon intuition or perception. But Hursthouse believes that such deontologists have a particular conception of what counts as an adequate normative ethics, namely one that provides adequate action-guidance. These deontologists hold that an adequate moral theory is one 'that yields a decision procedure which can be used to resolve conflicts or settle moral quandaries without recourse to moral wisdom'.[104] We have seen that act-utilitarians argue that their theory, with its single rule, provides just such a decision procedure. If one wants a moral theory that prescribes right action and ignores other morally important features, then act-utilitarianism is one to take seriously. O'Neill describes the SCT as 'an algorithm not just for some situations but for life'.[105]

Hursthouse believes that there are some deontologists who for one reason or another do not accept this algorithm as an appropriate test of adequacy. Kantians would probably reject it since, as O'Neill claims, Kant denies the possibility of such an algorithm. According to O'Neill, Kant held that 'every application of a rule would itself need supplementing with further rules'.[106] Other non-Kantian deontologists claim that the ability to recognize the morally important features of a concrete situation requires not only judgement but also 'moral sensitivity, perception, [and] imagination'.[107] Notably, according to Hursthouse this *is* moral wisdom. The result in the end is a division of opinion about the meaning of adequacy in relation to moral theories.

Deontology: Conclusions

I have noted several objections with deontological views that provide cause for concern. These include problems with the narrow framing and direction of deontological constraints, the lack of specific action-guidance until deontology's second premise (despite an assumption to the contrary), a lack of clarity regarding the distinction between intended and foreseen harm, problems with the nature and content of deontology's rules and problems inherent in relying on intuition to resolve the ranking of obligations, rules or principles.

Conclusions

I have examined forms of consequentialism and deontology and noted some of the common objections levelled at these obligation-based theories. Consequentialism makes the notion of the Right prior to the notion of the Good, while deontology views morality the other way around. However, both kinds of theory *over* focus on the role of moral obligations in morality. The notions of permission, prohibition and the aim to prescribe right action are held to be extremely important in determining the morally right and wrong action/omission. To this end, decision procedures are produced to resolve dilemmas. Both kinds of theory make assumptions concerning the nature of moral dilemmas, for instance, that they are *always* resolvable. Furthermore, the notion of moral remainder as discussed by Hursthouse is a very important topic, but one that is neglected by the vast majority of traditional obligation-based ethicists. It seems to me that there is nothing intrinsically about obligation-based theories that precludes the discussion of the role of emotions and feelings in morality. The traditional versions of obligation-based moral theories discussed in this chapter omit to explore too many morally important features; they are thus incomplete moral theories. Particularly with regard to failing to provide a rich and textured account of moral character, I conclude by agreeing with thinkers such as Rachels and Williams that these obligation-based moral theories are inadequate.

5
The Origins, Development and Tenets of Virtue Ethics

Introduction

I have critiqued obligation-based moral theories in general ethics and I have articulated several important flaws central to these theories. I concluded that consequentialism and deontology are incomplete and inadequate moral theories. In this chapter, I will examine virtue ethics, the moral theory that argues that the virtues are central to morality and to the aim of living a morally good life. First, I trace the origins and development of virtue ethics. I then identify four central tenets of virtue ethics and note the distinction between supplementary and strong forms of virtue ethics. Next, I examine Aristotle's virtue ethics. I then look more closely at virtue ethics' account of moral character and moral education. In the next chapter, I examine some common objections to virtue ethics.

The origins and development of virtue ethics

As noted in Chapter 3, ancient Greek ethics including the pre-Socratics but principally Socrates, Plato and Aristotle focused on the notions of the good life for man, human nature and the virtues. Despite moral philosophers such as Aquinas and Hume acknowledging the importance of the virtues in morality, virtue ethics as an alternative moral theory was not realized until its recent revival by Anscombe[1] in 1958. Virtue ethics now joins consequentialism (including utilitarianism) and deontology as an alternative moral theory. Anscombe argued that modern moral philosophy was bankrupt and misguided. She claimed that modern moral philosophy was grounded in the incoherent notion of a law, without a lawgiver. To virtue ethicists, this idea now makes no sense; neither do the related notions of obligation, duty, rightness and wrongness. Anscombe urged us to jettison the notions of 'right action' and 'morally right action', indeed the entire class of deontic notions. She claimed that things would be greatly improved if such notions were no longer used. Conduct in general or particular acts/omissions could be evaluated by using different aretaic (virtue and vice) terms such as 'dishonest', 'fair', 'kind' and 'unjust'. Instead of this flawed preoccupation with deontic theories and notions, Anscombe believed that the virtues should once again be the focus of ethics and she urged us to return to Aristotelian ethics.

The central tenets of virtue ethics

Critics allege that there is no such thing as a theory of virtue, meaning that all of the versions of virtue ethics are distinct and different. According to Rachels, there is 'no settled body of doctrine on which all these writers agree'.[2] Of course, it is possible to level this criticism at the many distinct versions of obligation-based moral theories. In its defence, the revival of virtue ethics started quite recently, and compared with obligation-based moral theories, virtue ethics is an immature and underdeveloped theory. With more scholarly work, I believe that virtue ethics will be clarified, developed and refined. What is not in doubt, however, is that versions of virtue ethics share a set of concerns that are largely ignored in obligation-based ethics. I shall use the term 'tenet' to describe these concerns because these mark out virtue ethics as a distinct moral theory and a credible alternative to consequentialism and deontology. I shall list four central tenets of virtue ethics:

1 It provides a detailed account of moral character;
2 It provides a rich account of moral goodness;
3 It provides a plausible account of moral education;
4 It provides a natural and convincing account of moral motivation.

Furthermore, several aspects of morality, while not solely connected to virtue ethics, have developed in part from examining the aims of moral theories and specifically, the relationship between 'right action' and 'good character'. An example of this is Hursthouse's three claims in relation to moral dilemmas that I discussed in Chapter 3. To recap: first, one should not assume that dilemmas are resolvable. Second, many dilemmas turn out to be 'irresolvable' or 'tragic'. Third, in all three types of dilemmas, it is morally appropriate for the moral agents involved to feel moral remainder. The latter refers to the feelings and emotions such as distress, remorse, guilt and regret that virtuous agents feel during and after their involvement in such distressing moral dilemmas. Moral remainder applies particularly to irresolvable and tragic dilemmas because the hurt and damage sustained in agents' lives is much more intense. Partly, as a consequence of Hursthouse's claims and partly because of virtue ethics' focus on the virtues and vices and the importance of human responsiveness and relationships, it seems to me that virtue ethics makes much more room for the role of feelings and emotions in the moral life than do the traditional accounts of consequentialism and deontology.

Virtue ethics: Nomenclature

I distinguish between supplementary and strong[3] (also called radical or free-standing) theories.

Supplementary virtue ethics

Supplementary theories view the virtues and a corresponding virtue ethics as requiring assistance from a version of obligation-based moral theories. This approach (also known as essentialism[4]) combines an account of right action provided by obligation-based ethics, for example, consequentialism or deontology, with an emphasis on moral character provided by the virtues and virtue ethics. The account of the virtues is offered as a supplement to an obligation-based theory of right action. Rachels[5] believes that this approach has much to recommend it.

Supplementary virtue ethics: Weak and moderate versions

Supplementary versions of virtue ethics can be further subdivided into those that hold that (a) obligations and right action are more important than the virtues and moral character in morality, and (b) the virtues and moral character are more important in morality than obligations and right action. The former can be called 'weak' and the latter 'moderate' versions of virtue ethics. In weak versions, the claim is that moral character is not as important as prescribing 'right action' and 'doing the right thing'; thus, while the virtues have a role to play in morality it is thought to be a rather unimportant one. This emphasis on 'right action' and revealing the morally correct decision is one of the core tenets of traditional accounts of obligation-based moral theories. Conversely, moderate versions of virtue ethics view morality the other way around claiming that moral character takes precedence over right action. Therefore, it is more important for people to cultivate and exercise the virtues, thus taking care of moral character rather than focusing on the idea of 'doing the right thing' although the latter point is where moral obligations remain implicated.

Supplementary virtue ethics in medicine: Pellegrino and Thomasma

Pellegrino and Thomasma's[6] version of virtue ethics in medicine is a supplementary theory. The authors regard moral principles as having greater moral force than the virtues. Moral obligations are held to be important to the moral conduct of physicians, and without such duties virtue ethics will be unable to adequately prescribe action-guidance for physicians. The major concern is that physicians might exercise the virtues of, for instance, honesty, justice and compassion and yet they might end up doing wrong actions. Pellegrino and Thomasma claim that there is a strong link between moral principles and corresponding virtues, each supplementing and informing the other.[7]

Supplementary and strong virtue ethics in nursing

Brody[8] published an influential article in 1988 in which she examined the role of caring and the virtues in nursing adults; I believe that this is a moderate version of virtue ethics. Examples of supplementary virtue ethics in mental health nursing are those of Lutzen and Barbosa da Silva[9] and McKie and Swinton.[10] I will not discuss the latter, but I note that while it is steeped in Aristotle and pays homage to MacIntyre (both of whom advocate a strong virtue ethics), McKie and Swinton's conception remains supplementary, albeit one that is perhaps moderate in terms of how important they view the importance of the virtues in moral decision-making. More recently, Begley[11] has critically examined the plausibility of a strong action-guiding version of virtue ethics for nursing practice and in particular, she picks up on Hursthouse's v-rules thesis. Begley believes that Hursthouse's claims regarding virtue ethics' provision for action-guidance challenges the common objection that virtue ethics lacks practical content and as such is of limited use in nursing ethics and nursing practice.

Lutzen and Barbosa da Silva's virtue ethics

Lutzen and Barbosa da Silva discuss the concept of virtue and the role of virtue ethics as a necessary but insufficient complement to rule-based ethics in psychiatric nursing. They claim that the relational aspects of nursing such as human interactions as well as moral principles and rules need emphasizing. For the authors, moral motivation, which has largely been ignored in traditional obligation-based ethics, is necessary in a moral activity such as nursing:

> Virtue ethics serves as a necessary complement in an ethical framework for health care practice with regard to the moral agent as such (the kind of person he/she ought to be) and the motivation for obeying or following a given moral obligation or duty in concrete situations.[12]

The authors argue that virtues enable the nurse to evaluate a moral dilemma, identify all the morally relevant features and then apply the appropriate moral rules and principles to the dilemma. Both intellectual and moral virtues are needed 'for the realization of various kinds of duties or moral obligations'.[13] Further, it is necessary to have practical wisdom as this allows for the 'realization of the other virtues'.[14] The authors argue that besides the theoretical knowledge possessed by the nurse, it is necessary to ask: 'What kind of person one is as a moral agent.'[15] This supplementary approach has its merits, for example, at least the authors recognize the importance of the virtues in moral decision-making in nursing. It is, however, unclear whether the authors would argue for a weak or moderate position. My view is that this version represents a weak version of virtue ethics. Virtue is held to be necessary, but not sufficient to morality in nursing. The authors essentially claim that virtues help to provide the right motivation for the nurse in order to decide which moral rules to obey and follow. The authors clearly believe that nurses need nursing knowledge and moral principles/rules to make the 'right moral decision' or the 'morally right decision'. However, I think that the authors confuse two ways in which these terms can be used, which I credited to the work of Hursthouse in Chapter 3. I shall present a clinical situation that will be used to bring out this confusion: Mary, a 65-year-old female is diagnosed with a primary endogenous major depressive disorder. She has had electroconvulsive therapy (ECT) with good results in the past. On this occasion though, after the first two treatments, she refuses to have a third. She is 'reassured' into having another treatment by the charge nurse, despite saying: 'I don't want another treatment … I'm afraid. Don't make me go.' After having this and subsequent treatments, she recovered and was discharged.[16] Suppose that this is a resolvable dilemma: act x is to coerce Mary to have ECT, while act y is to respect her wish to refuse ECT. It is thought that act x should be carried out because it is more beneficial than y. This can then be called a 'right moral decision' or the 'morally right decision' given the worse option of *y*. However, a second way in which these terms can be used refers to a morally good deed, for example, when a person displays the virtues and performs an admirable act, one that others praise. This meaning cannot be applied to act *x* – helping to force Mary into having ECT is not a virtuous, morally admirable or morally good deed. This confusion is a problem that affects obligation-based moral theories in general. But it is also, in my view, the flaw in supplementary virtue ethics. I understand why some ethicists wish to develop supplementary accounts of virtue ethics. For example, it might be thought that adding in the virtues will ensure that moral character is not neglected. But as long as virtue is conceived in terms of helping persons (nurses) to decide upon which moral obligations to act from, then introducing the virtues will not reveal the confusion between the two meanings of 'right moral decision/morally right decision'. Irrespective of whether the theory is weak or moderate this confusion will continue. The implication is that the virtues will only be allowed to operate as a necessary component of nursing ethics, as a way of identifying the correct moral obligations to use in particular situations. In this way, the focus will remain on the first meaning of 'right moral decision/morally right decision'. But the second meaning of these phrases, i.e., a morally good, admirable and virtuous deed will not be appreciated.

Strong virtue ethics

Strong versions of virtue ethics (also known as eliminatism[17]) include Aristotle, MacIntyre and Hursthouse. Some of Hursthouse's claims were presented in Chapter 3 and 4 and her influence is felt throughout this book, while Chapter 9 is devoted to MacIntyre's virtue ethics. These ethicists hold that virtue ethics and the virtues are capable of doing all the work of ethics. Rachels calls this 'an independent theory of ethics that is complete in itself'.[18] For strong virtue ethicists, one's moral character, moral motivations and the justification of acts/omissions are couched solely in the virtues. These ethicists reject the use of deontic language such as 'right' and 'wrong' and are influenced by Anscombe who urged us to jettison all deontic notions from ethics. Instead, strong virtue ethicists would justify, for instance, not bullying someone, not because it is 'wrong', 'unethical' or 'it breaks the moral rule "do not harm others"', but because 'it is cruel'. Instead of deontic terms, the language of the virtues and vices is employed.

Aristotle's virtue ethics

In this section, I examine Aristotle's conception of ethics drawn from Books one and two of *The Nicomachean Ethics*. I do so for two reasons: first, Aristotle is a pivotal philosopher in the history of virtue ethics and has influenced several contemporary moral philosophers including Hursthouse and MacIntyre; and second, this section helps to provide the philosophical foundation for Chapter 9 on MacIntyre's virtue ethics.

Aristotle on the good life

For the ancient Greeks, ethics was viewed as a component of politics and the focus was very much on protecting states. Deontic notions had not been conceptualized in ancient Greece, thus ethics was not concerned with moral obligation. Instead Aristotle was concerned with questions such as 'What sort of people do we have to be if we are to live the good life?' What does Aristotle mean by the good life? To understand this, one needs to examine Aristotle's account of human nature. The opening words of *The Nicomachean Ethics* are:

> Every art and every inquiry, and similarly every action and pursuit, is thought to aim at some good; and for this reason the good has rightly been declared to be that at which all things aim.[19]

It is noted, however, that some pursuits, for example, child abuse, war and terrorism aim at evil or causing great harm. Despite this, Aristotle believed that actions and pursuits aimed at good. One might choose one good, say, friendship over another, say, the pleasures of food, where neither holds priority. In this way, it is possible to go on *ad infinitum*. Aristotle thought that there must be a chief good, one that is chosen for its own sake. All moral inquiry sought to investigate the nature of this chief good. For Aristotle, it was important for everyone to understand the need to pursue this chief good. However Aristotle's argument is circular. He believed that to know what the good consists of one must have had the 'right' moral education and the 'right' character. In other words, one must be virtuous to know what the good consists of. But presumably one must know what the good consists of to be virtuous.

Eudaimonia

For Aristotle, the chief good for man was 'eudaimonia'. There is disagreement over the precise meaning of this term. Ross[20] and Benn[21] translate this as 'happiness'. However, others use 'flourishing'. Which term is more appropriate? For many 'happiness' conjures up the satisfaction of physical and psychological needs although some people may be more myopic on this and view happiness solely in terms of satisfying physical needs. Perhaps 'flourishing' suggests a more overall state of affairs; when one flourishes one fares well and one's life goes well. Perhaps to fare well, we require more than just the satisfaction of our needs, perhaps our interests need to be promoted too. This description could also apply to well-being, a term that many obligation-based ethicists are fond of using. Perhaps when my interests are promoted, then my well-being is promoted too. Happiness and well-being could therefore be synonymous. But is flourishing the same as well-being? Both terms suggest an organism's overall state of harmony. To fare well, one's interests and needs need to be met, perhaps flourishing emphasizes non-physical needs such as emotional and spiritual needs. This debate could be discussed at length without drawing firm conclusions. However, in relation to the translation of eudaimonia it is plausible to suggest that well-being and happiness are synonymous and that flourishing shares some of these characteristics too. Benn remarks that eudaimonia is not, like euphoria, a psychological state. Instead it refers to one's life faring well. If I am faring well, then I flourish. Will I always be happy when I flourish? Will there be moments of unhappiness even when I reckon that, on the whole, I am doing well? Of course there will be. A typical day in the life of Robert (the charity worker in Chapter 3) will contain moments of sadness, distress and unhappiness. Nevertheless, he fares well and succeeds in his role. A connection exists 'between feeling happy and having your life go well'.[22] But there might be moments when one's life is going well on the whole and yet one experiences sadness or misery from a myriad of sources and for many reasons. Given the diversity of our interests and needs, there will be 'more and less fulfilling ways of going about these things'.[23] However, one is led very sharply into the moral high ground if one attempts to distinguish between these kinds of activities. So far in this book, instead of using the term 'flourishing', I have used the phrases 'to fare well', 'faring well' and 'one's life going well'. Both 'flourishing' and 'to fare well' form part of a typical conception of flourishing; I refer the reader to philosophical literature on the latter notion.[24] In this chapter, I use 'flourishing' because this is the usual translation of Aristotle's 'eudaimonia'. But in my view 'faring well' and 'flourishing' are equivalent.

What does flourishing comprise?

For Aristotle, this concerns the function of the organism or object in question; everything, whether a spoon, pencil or man had a characteristic function or activity. For instance, the function of a knife is to cut. Aristotle thought that the *characteristic* function of man cannot be biological living because this applies to a whole range of animals and plants. For such a function or activity to be characteristic of man, it needed to be unique to humans. In his view, this was the life of reason. In his words, this rational element is

> activity of soul exhibiting excellence, and if there be more than one excellence, in accordance with the best and the most complete.[25]

According to Aristotle, man would flourish as long as he met the function of reason and crucially, it was important that man carried out his function excellently. But what conception of excellence or good did Aristotle have in mind? On human good he wrote: 'Human good turns out to be an activity of soul exhibiting excellence'[26] (although this sounds almost identical to his definition of reason, above). For Aristotle, every human activity has an appropriate excellence and the aim for man was to carry out these activities in an excellent manner.

Goodness and function

For Aristotle there was a tight relationship between being a good person and human function. For a person to flourish, one must live in accordance with the distinctive function of man. As noted, Aristotle believed this was excellence in reason; man lived well if he lived according to a rational principle. For Aristotle the best[27] life was one of pure theoretical contemplation, i.e., the life of a philosopher. Aristotle believed that the essence of being a good man was the ability to think well. This approach has advantages for the justification of morality, especially the desire to make it more objective. Moral truth becomes a naturalistic truth in the sense that one can empirically assess (by using the special senses) whether x is good or not. One can watch man to see if he is living according to his function. Or one can observe a boat to see whether it moves smoothly over water and floats; if it does, it is a good boat. However, if it sinks then it is not a good boat. This is true even if it looks fabulous; it is not a good boat because it has failed to meet its function.[28]

The use of 'good'

The above discussion introduces an important point made by Benn[29] about the use of 'good'. When one considers 'the QE2 was a good ship', one does not mean *both* good *and* a ship. Rather one means 'the QE2 was good *as* a ship'. Further, if one says about Robert the charity worker in Chapter 3 that 'he is a good man', one does not mean *both* good *and* a man, but good *as* a man. This is because goodness is related to the degree that one succeeds in discharging one's function; this suggests a crude form of functionalism.[30] To speak of 'goodness in men' means that one compares men and makes a judgement. According to Benn, one means something like 'Jack is a good man, *as far as men go*' [my italics]. 'Good' is not only used here as a term of approval, it is also a descriptive term. How does this lead to a more objective ethics? Benn responds:

> If we can discern man's function, and discern who is living according to it, we have an objective, descriptive answer to questions about goodness in men.[31]

According to Aristotle's theory, if John performs an action that inclines him towards his function as a man, then it is a right action and *vice versa*. If human goodness is construed in this way, then one negates the use of action-guiding principles and properties proposed by consequentialists and deontologists. Instead one needs to examine men in action and their goodness can be then evaluated.

Hitting the right mark: The doctrine of the mean

As noted in Chapter 3, according to Aristotle virtue is not a passion or emotion nor is it a faculty such as the capacity to feel anger or fear. Rather, virtue is a state of character. For Aristotle, it is possible to take more, less or an equal amount of everything, 'and the equal [the mean] is an intermediate between excess and defect'.[32] This is Aristotle's 'doctrine of the mean'. Take courage, for example. Here, the excess is rashness, while the deficiency is cowardice. A necessary quality of virtue on Aristotle's account is that it must aim at the intermediate. Aristotle qualifies this to mean 'moral virtue' for this 'is concerned with passions and actions, and in these there is excess, defect and the intermediate'.[33] Aristotle realizes, however, that it is not easy to be good; he believed: 'In everything it is no easy task to find the middle.'[34] How should one go about achieving the virtuous mean? Determining the mean is not reducible to abstract, specific moral rules or general moral principles such as 'maximise the good' or 'always treat others as ends'. Aristotle claimed that it is best if one tries to disregard or dismiss aiming at pleasure because this is usually a partial judgement. He held that once this is done, 'we are less likely to go astray ... [and] ... we shall best be able to hit the mean'.[35] The difficult process of determining the mean does not depend on reasoning; notably, this claim might appear obscure coming from someone who placed such a firm emphasis on this faculty. Nevertheless, Aristotle claimed that perception (not reasoning) determined the mean. This was because the senses discover what is going on around us, and perception via the senses enables one to take stock of particular facts and circumstances needed to hit the mean. Despite realizing the difficulty of hitting the mean, Aristotle lays down demanding criteria before people can achieve true virtue. For example, he held that giving away one's money was in terms of moral goodness insufficient. But,

> to do this to the right person, to the right extent, at the right time, with the right motive, and in the right way, *that* is not for everyone, nor is it easy; wherefore goodness is both rare and laudable and noble.[36]

I am uncertain whether the above stringent criteria could be met by anyone. Further, would one wish someone to be like this? The use of 'right' also makes for an incredibly subjective checklist. For example, one might get the motive and amount 'right'. But who counts as 'the right person'? Aristotle might have thought it virtuous to give his money away to a friend, another Athenian gentleman. But given his criteria, I doubt he would think it virtuous to give away his money to a beggar who would more than not benefit greatly from it.

Aristotle believed that becoming virtuous was not a matter of learning moral rules. Instead, it required the cultivation of certain dispositions and the education of one's desires. Aristotle viewed desires as 'irrational elements in the soul'.[37] While our desires might not in themselves realize a rational principle, when one's desires respond to a rational principle moral virtue is acquired. Reason need not ignore or override desire; indeed desire was the major motive behind all actions. On moral motivation, Aristotle held:

> Actions, then, are just and temperate when they are such as the just or the temperate man would do; but it is not the man who does these that is just and temperate, but the man who also does them *as* just and temperate men do them.[38]

Aristotle thus makes a distinction between 'acting virtuously, and acting in conformity with virtue'.[39] He claimed that the exercise of the virtues must represent a person's true or real character; in other words, this must be second nature. For Aristotle, persons' dispositions to make the right choices are displayed in their desires. It was, therefore, crucial that the education of character was taught so that these dispositions are acquired. Aristotle realized that this is not an innate or natural process; it must begin in early childhood if she/he is to become a virtuous adult. In this sense, acquiring virtue is similar to any discipline requiring a certain skill such as playing chess or learning to play a musical instrument where both require plenty of practice. One acts, firstly, as if one already possesses the disposition in question. This involves training oneself to do virtuous deeds. In time, one gains the necessary dispositions to habitually achieve these things in accordance with reason and the good life.

There was no room in Aristotle's ethics for several common contemporary virtues, for example, kindness, compassion and honesty. Instead the so-called cardinal virtues of justice, courage, wisdom and temperance played a prominent role in his account of the moral life. These virtues were needed to enable human flourishing. For example, courage was needed to deal with dangerous and frightening challenges, while temperance was important because

> the ability to forswear or postpone the gratification of desire is essential to getting what we really want, and to lasting happiness.[40]

Different historical eras value different virtues. For example, Aristotle valued pride (or megalopsuchia), but pride was condemned by medieval Christian philosophers as one of the 'seven deadly sins'. And while Aristotle condemned boastfulness, he did not value humility. Despite this, several thinkers such as Hursthouse and Benn believe that one can derive much useful guidance on the moral life from Aristotle's ethics.

Objections to Aristotle's ethics

There are several established criticisms of Aristotle's ethics. First, it should not be assumed that man has a function, i.e., man might not be 'for' something. Merely because man does things that are in some way guided by reasoning does not in itself mean that this is man's function. People have various interests and needs and participate in a myriad of activities that reflect their values. However, these values do not necessarily imply a function. In other words, 'can' does not mean 'should'. In Benn's words:

> The mere fact that there are certain things he can do and sometimes does, is a poor ground for thinking this is what he *should* be doing.[41]

It is not clear that man has a specific function. Therefore, it is unclear that the good life should be discerned as the fulfilment of such a function. Even if we accept that the good life is related in some way to human reason, it remains problematic to identify this 'completely with the *moral* life'.[42] However, Benn concedes that

> there is *some* connection between the flourishing of our most distinctive qualities, and the possession of moral virtue.[43]

The point is that humans display many excellences besides moral ones including artistic and creative talents, social skills, beauty, physical strength and mental determination. All of these qualities are valued by people, and some of these qualities are also unique to humans and as such, have a right to define the function of man. In response to this objection, it is possible for contemporary Aristotelians to accept the claim that denies creatures have a purpose and still accept other claims made by Aristotle. For example, eyes have evolved over many millions of years; they exist and they enable their bearers to see. However, as Benn claims, they did not develop literally in order to see. A purpose does not necessarily lie behind the process of evolution by natural selection. However, eyes do *enable* their bearers to see and in contrast, eyes that do not enable vision are damaged or defective. Supporters of Aristotle's functionalism may ask: 'What do eyes do best?' The answer presumably is 'seeing'. Advocates of Aristotle might then ask: 'Is there something that humans do best?' For some people, the answer to this will be 'reasoning'; so for these people, people will flourish – fare well and lead good lives – if they reason well.

The second criticism alleges that even if we accept that man does have a function, it still does not follow that this function (whichever activity is chosen) is unique to him. Even if no other creature lives according to reason, it is implausible to claim that this is what man is *for* and that doing this will ensure his goodness. In response to this criticism, perhaps the meaning of 'a rational principle' could be understood too narrowly. There are many forms of reasoning. Words such as 'rational' and 'thinking' cover a multitude of these forms that include practical reasoning, theoretical contemplation, perception and the experiencing of emotions. It is difficult to sharply define these examples of reasoning; all involve to some degree an element of understanding. Furthermore, it is unhelpful to make crude generalizations. For example, in claiming 'emotions do not involve reasoning' one makes an error because there is a rational element to experiencing emotions. Indeed everything we do involves some form of reasoning. Although other creatures feel and perceive, humans do so in a way that *is* unique. I concur with Benn who claims that all aspects of human life are affected by the process of reasoning (the latter understood in broad terms).

Third, let us accept that man participates in activities unique to him such as sports.[44] Why is the life of reason chosen ahead of these other unique human activities? In reply, one might claim that *all* of these activities are rational, i.e., they all involve some form of reasoning. One cannot, for example, participate in sport without reasoning. This appears true. But now one is left with an empty definition of 'reasoning' because the range of activities is all-inclusive and too broad to be insightful. Instead, one could limit the sorts of activities that one believes reflect man's rational function such as philosophical enquiry. But besides these rational activities, many other activities presumably thought 'less rational' than philosophical enquiry will remain, such as playing football. Since it is claimed that other creatures cannot engage in philosophical enquiry or football, why is one of these other activities not held to be the chief function? A fourth criticism charges that Aristotle is elitist when he claims that the life of contemplation is the *best* sort of life for a human to lead. It is possible to lead a good life by interacting with others, by helping and caring about others and by displaying different forms and degrees of reasoning such as practical reasoning. Social elitism, slavery and sexism lie at the core of Aristotle's ethics; women in particular were treated unjustly by the standards of modernity. Hursthouse refers to these values as 'deplorable'.[45] Only males of high social standing, in effect, Athenian gentlemen could achieve full virtue. Contemporary virtue ethicists, for example, Hursthouse[46] and MacIntyre[47] are referred to as neo-Aristotelians because they have rejected these outdated and unjust views and adapted their own versions of virtue ethics accordingly. Benn claims that these criticisms should not detract from discussion of the remainder of Aristotle's ethics. He thinks it consistent to deny Aristotle's outdated and unjust ideas on slavery, women and social hierarchy and still accept other plausible strands in his virtue ethics.

A fifth and perhaps more notable objection to Aristotelian ethics questions the connection between the moral life and the sort of life that might benefit an individual. This is not as close and substantial as Aristotle supposed. One is thus led to ask: 'Does it pay to lead the moral life?'[48] It is possible for one to fare well without being virtuous. For instance, Benn mentions the wealthy aesthete

> who lacks a social conscience, and surrounds himself with fine things and refined human company.[49]

I shall now describe virtue ethics' account of moral character including its response to the impartialism advocated by utilitarianism. I then look at Hursthouse's account of action-guidance, which she frames in terms of 'v-rules'. I end this chapter by briefly considering virtue ethics and moral education.

Virtue ethics and moral character

As noted in Chapter 4, consequentialism and deontology, respectively, over focus on the consequences of acts/omissions or the nature and content of moral obligations. At least in the traditional versions of these theories, questions concerning people's moral characters and their moral lives are neglected. To rectify this serious omission, one of the main concerns of virtue ethics is to provide a richer more textured account of moral character. Virtue ethics gives special consideration to people's character traits, both the virtues and vices (as discussed in Chapter 3). Virtue ethicists are primarily concerned with the kind of person one is. One of the requirements of a virtue-based approach to morality is self-reflection; for example, on what kind of person one is and on the sort of life one wishes to lead. Important questions include 'How can I be a morally good (excellent) person? What does acting in a certain way such as honestly say about me as a person? And how ought I to respond to this person's interests and needs? In an attempt to derive some action-guidance regarding the general question 'What sort of person should I be?', one can ask another more specific question 'What would a virtuous – for example, honest – person do in these circumstances?' Virtuous people will be repelled at the thought of vicious deeds and take great pleasure in carrying out virtuous deeds. This can be sharply contrasted with Kant's ideas on moral worth because for him, pleasure was unimportant when carrying out acts.[50] Back to Stocker's example for a moment (in Chapter 3), while one might have admiration for people who act *solely* from a sense of duty, 'we tend to think better of agents who like to do what they ought, because their good deeds express their real character'.[51] The role of motives is also crucially important in virtue ethics. An important criticism of obligation-based moral theories is that they provide a hard and inflexible duty-based account of moral motivation, which does not accurately reflect the lives of humans (see the discussion based on Stocker's example in Chapter 3). Moreover, both consequentialism and deontology are criticized because they fail to provide a rigorous account of the distinctiveness of persons and the significance of relationships in human life.[52] Slote[53] is a virtue ethicist who believes that virtues provide one with the reasons and motives for acts, thoughts and feelings. Slote believes that the virtues are admirable character traits that form one's reason for cultivating and exercising the virtues. His version of virtue ethics is unusual because it is not grounded in Aristotle; instead Slote's theory is derived from the moral sentimentalism of Hume and Martineau. In Slote's theory, 'caring' is the one foundational virtue. 'Caring' is admirable and this claim does not depend upon, for example, the consequences of caring. For Slote, virtues *are* motives; for example, kindness is a morally admirable trait, a virtue and it also serves as the motive for action. The rightness of an act on Slote's view derives from the nature of the motive behind it; if a person carries out a deed from the motive of kindness, then it is a kind deed and as such, it is a morally good (and right) deed.[54]

For some people, actions and beliefs are either right or wrong. Some actions and beliefs are more absolute than others, i.e., actions and beliefs are either absolutely right or absolutely wrong. For example, 'value human life' and 'do not murder' are for many people examples of beliefs that are absolutely (always) right, while 'harm children' is for many people an example of a belief that is absolutely (always) wrong. Rather than evaluating these beliefs from an act perspective, virtue ethics can provide an insight into the character and motives of people who commit such acts or hold such beliefs. Instead of asking 'How is the world improved or made worse by such and such an action?' the virtue ethicist is concerned about 'What the doing of this action would reveal about the one who does it?'[55] For example, would an honest or compassionate person do such a thing? Or are these the acts or thoughts of a dishonest or cruel agent? According to Benn, this way of reasoning leads us to

a set of moral concerns that is more plausible than anything that can be delivered by purely action-based accounts.[56]

Virtue ethics and impartialism

In Chapter 4, it was noted that act consequentialism results in conflicts with some deep moral intuitions such as the wrongness of murder, slavery and torture. Consequentialism in particular utilitarianism advocates impartialism and yet some moral intuitions support partialism towards one's loved ones. The virtue ethicist, however, does not face the stringent problem of impartialism. Instead virtue ethics can accommodate the notion of partialism quite easily. Rather than asking what the abstract notion of impartiality and partiality mean, virtue ethics seeks to understand the virtues involved in forming and sustaining close relationships with others. Virtue ethics also aims to understand how one virtue, say, honesty relates to another, say, compassion.

Virtue ethics and moral education

Obligation-based moral theories ask: 'Is this action morally right or wrong?' In response, one typically thinks of reasons for and against doing the act. One often believes that the act with the best (most convincing) reasons should be carried out. If an obligation-based ethics is adopted, these reasons will be related to (a) maximizing utility or at least producing good rather than bad consequences and (b) abiding by moral obligations, rules or principles. There is, however, a third source of knowledge that people can utilize when they want to know what to do. This is to seek the moral guidance of someone else; someone whom one believes is morally wiser than oneself, someone whom one admires. Indeed, the main 'method' of teaching the virtues is by instruction from others, observing other people who are virtuous and admired and aiming to be like these people. Virtue ethics recognizes that these points are important and crucial in people's moral lives. However, obligation-based ethics appears to ignore this option. Indeed, asking others for their view is almost regarded as morally deficient. In my experience, many people seek guidance from 'wiser' people including close friends, relatives and colleagues. This fact is particularly important for virtue ethicists who believe that it should be accepted and endorsed for what it is, namely, a claim about something that does happen. People are a valuable resource of knowledge, ideas and views that are sometimes needed when one really does not know what to do. Of course, this is rejected by obligation-based ethics because these theories hold that all dilemmas can be resolved as long as the person acts in accordance with its obligations, rules and principles. But this fails to represent the moral life in realistic terms, i.e., complex, multifaceted, richly textured and full of moral confusion.

Conclusions

In this chapter, I have examined the origins and development of virtue ethics and explained the difference between supplementary and strong versions of virtue ethics, and I described Aristotle's ethics as an example of the latter. Merits of virtue ethics include its rich portrayal of moral character and its emphasis on moral education. Of course, like other alternative moral theories, virtue ethics has come under attack from critics. In Chapter 6, I will examine some of the common objections levelled at virtue ethics.

6
Common Objections to Virtue Ethics

Introduction

In this chapter I will identify and examine several common criticisms levelled at virtue ethics. One of the aims of this chapter is to consider whether a strong, i.e., action-guiding version of virtue ethics is plausible.

Hursthouse on action-guidance and the v-rules

In Chapter 4, I noted Hursthouse's work on moral dilemmas and the idea of moral remainder. In *On Virtue Ethics*, Hursthouse also responds to the common criticism that virtue ethics cannot provide a person with adequate action-guidance. Obligation-based ethicists charge that the virtuous agent will have no idea what to do in particular dilemmas because they argue that virtue ethics fails to come up with any rules for conduct. Hursthouse believes that this is wrong. In her view, people have access to a whole range of virtues and as I noted in Chapter 3, within the structure of these virtues and vices there is considerable moral guidance. For example, the virtues include compassion, honesty and patience. The virtuous person would, therefore, characteristically be compassionate, true to her word and patient in the circumstances. Virtuous persons would not be non-compassionate (or cruel), lie or impatient. Hursthouse believes that despite one's own initial uncertainty, it is possible to have a very good idea of what the virtuous person would do. For example, Hursthouse asks:

> Would she lie in her teeth to acquire an unmerited advantage? No, for that would be both dishonest and unjust ... Might she keep a death-bed promise even though living people would benefit from its being broken? Yes, for she is true to her word. And so on.[1]

Furthermore, Hursthouse believes that virtue ethics 'comes up with a large number of rules'.[2] It clearly gives one prescriptions for action, for example, 'do what is *honest*', 'do what is *just*' and 'do what is *compassionate*'. But virtue ethics also tells one what not to do: 'each vice [is] a prohibition – do not do what is dishonest, uncharitable, mean'. Hursthouse calls these the v-rules (I believe that this refers to 'virtuous' or 'vicious' rules, but this is not made clear). In developing this thesis about the v-rules, Hursthouse demonstrates that virtue ethics *does* present an account of right action that includes rules thus denying the common criticism that it fails to. This criticism is grounded in the common view that virtue ethics is about 'Being' rather than 'Doing'. It is more accurate to claim that 'virtue ethics focuses on Being i.e., moral character but does not do so at the expense of Doing, i.e. action guidance'. Because virtue ethics provides rules for guidance, it is now possible to rebut the claim that for virtue ethics to work adequately it needs to be supplemented with other deontic rules. Given that virtue ethics provides action-guidance, are there other reasons for thinking that it cannot tell people what to do? Perhaps the v-rules of virtue ethics are the wrong sort of rules? Rules like 'Do what is honest' and 'Do not do what is unkind' are like the rule 'Do what the virtuous person would do'. Hursthouse believes that the v-rules provide a different sort of action-guidance than that supplied by the rules of deontology and the one rule of act-utilitarianism. More specifically, Hursthouse believes that the v-rules 'are couched in terms, or concepts, that are certainly "evaluative" in *some* sense, or senses, of that difficult word'.[3] It appears that deontologists are discontent with the rule 'Do not kill' as they have refined it to include more sophisticated and evaluative terms such as 'Do not murder', 'Do not kill the innocent' and 'Do not kill unjustly' (although as Hursthouse notes, the latter is a specific form of v-rule). Deontologists might argue that the v-rules are inferior to their own rules when it comes to the moral education and guidance of children. In the case of children, 'the simple rules we learnt at our mother's knee are indispensable'.[4] The v-rules are 'thick' concepts in the sense that they are complex and sophisticated notions to pick up on. This is so for adults, but at least they are capable of rigorous thinking regarding what constitutes harming someone or promoting someone's well-being. This process will be more difficult for children and will depend upon their age and degree of physical, mental and moral maturity. Some v-rules including 'act charitably' and 'don't act unjustly' might be regarded as inappropriate for use with children because as Hursthouse notes: '[these thick concepts are] Far too thick for a child to grasp'.[5] Hursthouse believes that this objection – the v-rules are inadequate in providing guidance for children – is slightly different from the general critical claim that the v-rules do not provide action-guidance. It is more specific and concerns

> a condition of adequacy that any normative ethics must meet, namely that such an ethics must not only come up with action guidance for a clever rational adult, but also generate some account of moral education, of how one generation teaches the next what they should do.[6]

According to Hursthouse, there are two reasons why this criticism is false. First, she holds that the claim that toddlers are taught only deontological rules is wrong. She thinks that sentences such as 'Be *kind* to your brother, he's only little' and 'Don't be so *mean*, so *greedy*' are taught to children on a regular basis. However, she admits that while 'fair' and 'unfair' are taught, 'just' and 'unjust' are for some reason not. Second, Hursthouse believes that it is unnecessary for a virtue ethicist to deny significant deontological rules such as 'Do not lie' and 'Keep promises'. While she thinks it is wrong to define a virtuous agent as one who acts in accordance with deontological rules, it is perhaps an understandable mistake to make because of the obvious connection between the rule about not lying and the need to cultivate and exercise the virtue of honesty. It should be clear by now that distinctions between deontological moral rules and the virtues concern motives, ends and value. Implicated here is the acknowledgement that on the one hand, deontologists think it sufficient to teach a rule prohibiting lying, whereas on the other hand virtue ethicists 'want to emphasize the fact that, if children are to be taught to be honest, they must be taught to love and prize the truth'.[7] But according to Hursthouse, this end will not be realized via the deontological method. I agree with Hursthouse's point and it is an important one because virtue ethicists do not have to deny the usefulness of teaching children deontological moral rules. In summary, Hursthouse argues convincingly that virtue ethics comes up with rules for action – the v-rules. These include 'Be honest' and 'Do as the compassionate person would'. Moreover, virtue ethicists can also accept and accommodate the deontologist's familiar rules; certainly these rules, for example, 'Do not lie' need not be rejected. The distinction between the two is concerned with their different moral foundations. For example, deontology states that lying is wrong because it violates the rule 'Do not lie'; therefore lying is morally prohibited. On the virtue ethics view, however, people should not lie because it would be dishonest and dishonesty is a vice.

What is virtue ethics?

A second common criticism of virtue ethics is that virtue ethicists are unable to come up with a simple short answer to the question: 'What is virtue ethics?' (Although it seems that no one is bothered that this is also the case with deontology and utilitarianism.) Nevertheless, this objection is levelled at virtue ethicists as if it is a flaw in the theory itself that is somehow meant to make virtue ethics less plausible. In response to this criticism, Hursthouse believes that it is hard to describe virtue ethics in broad terms 'to get all virtue ethicists in' and at the same time, describe it 'sufficiently tight to keep all deontologists and utilitarians out'.[8] She thinks that this challenge is excessive. It is, I think, unfair because if virtue ethicists could do this then they would be unique among ethicists. The majority of individuals interested in moral philosophy simply do not know much about virtue ethics. This is one reason why the non-proponents of virtue ethics want it explained in just a few sentences. This is in contrast to the familiarity evident towards deontology and utilitarianism, theories that are usually taught in undergraduate philosophy courses (and in nursing education, there is evidence to suggest that consequentialism and deontology dominate the teaching of ethics).[9] Hursthouse would probably agree with my claim that virtue ethics is not taught as widely as the traditional obligation-based moral theories. As more thinkers become aware of virtue ethics and develop their understanding of it, it is likely that further consensus will be reached on its central tenets, aims and objectives.

Is strong virtue ethics a viable view?

Typically, obligation-based ethicists believe that a strong version of virtue ethics is implausible. Moral philosophers who accept the importance of the virtues in morality include Rachels;[10] however, he also believes that strong virtue ethics is not a viable view. Rachels accepts that theories that emphasize right action usually neglect the importance of moral character in the moral lives of agents. Virtue ethics, irrespective of its form, focuses upon moral character. But as Rachels reminds us:

> Moral problems are frequently about what we should *do*. It is not obvious how, according to virtue ethics, we should go about deciding what to do.[11]

Rachels believes that this strong approach is unnecessary; instead he believes that one could retain the notions of 'morally right' and 'right action', but interpret these from within the virtue ethics framework. However, it appears that Rachels has not conceived the action-guidance derivable from the virtues and vices in the way that Hursthouse has done. I believe that Hursthouse's v-rules thesis provides a plausible and satisfactory response to the common charge that virtue ethics cannot tell people what to do. We need to imagine virtuous people and ask, for example, 'Aunt Daisy is really *kind*, I wonder what she would do in this situation?' Instead of thinking in broad terms, i.e., encompassing all the virtues together, it is preferable to take one virtue at a time and think about what each separately entails. For instance, how should I act, think and feel if I wish to be *honest*?

Deontic versus aretaic language

In everyday life, there are numerous common moral rules[12] and principles, some stricter and weightier than others. For example, 'Do not harm the innocent', 'Tell the truth' and 'Don't break promises'. Such moral rules and principles are considered indispensable by many deontologists. The criticism is that the content of these rules and principles cannot be completely understood simply by reference to a specific virtue. In Benn's words:

> The concept of the virtues makes little sense apart from the idea that a virtuous individual is disposed to do the right things – and we seem to need some other account that can tell us what the right things are.[13]

This objection is basically saying that 'virtue-talk' cannot replace 'action-talk'. For many people, the concepts of 'right' and 'wrong' action are so important in morality that one should not as Anscombe[14] suggests jettison them. Contrast this to the virtuous person: a virtuous person is disposed to think virtuously, i.e., in terms of those virtues she cultivates. Further, she is disposed to do virtuous deeds, i.e., act from the virtues. Strong virtue ethicists do not use deontic language such as 'right action' or 'morally wrong action'. Instead, they use the language of specific virtues. For instance, instead of referring to someone as 'virtuous' one should be more accurate and use the relevant virtue, for example, 'John is a *just* man' or 'Mary is a *patient* lady'. In this way, one gets a much better, more detailed picture of the kind of people John and Mary are. Furthermore, instead of using deontic language such as 'right' and 'wrong', virtue ethicists refer to one's acts by using aretaic terms such as 'John (and Mary) act *well*' or conversely concerning someone who has exercised the vice of dishonesty, 'he acts *badly*'.

The problem of incompleteness

Related to the plausibility of strong virtue ethics, Rachels[15] identifies a problem concerning the sufficiency of virtue ethics. He asks: 'Is the virtue theorists' explanation of what we ought to do sufficient?' He believes that the virtue ethicists' explanation is incomplete. Take honesty as an example. The strong virtue ethicist tells us to be honest because it is a moral excellence that will help both the possessor and the benefactor to fare well in life (note that I am talking about faring well and leading good lives in a moral sense). Conversely, being dishonest is a vice that interferes with how humans are able to get on in life. As noted, people who cultivate the virtues are worthy of admiration and praise, while those who cultivate the vices are worthy of nothing less than moral repugnance. Probably the largest group of people are those who fail to realize the importance of the virtues and therefore do not cultivate them. However, if these people do not cultivate the vices then the moral assessment of these people is more difficult; one would need to know what kind of people, on the whole, they are.

What do the virtues entail?

Another related problem is the difficulty in knowing what a specific virtue entails. For instance, what precisely does it mean to be honest? I examined this type of question in Chapter 3, but since it is a criticism levelled at virtue ethics I shall look at it again. The supposed difficulty in answering this question is one reason why Rachels thinks deontological rules are important in morality. According to him, the response to 'Why shouldn't I lie?' needs to be more than 'because it goes against the character trait of honesty'. Why is it better to have the trait of honesty rather than its opposite? Convincing reasons are needed to show why it is morally preferable to be honest rather than dishonest (to be kind rather than unkind and so on). In response to this, Rachels writes:

> Possible answers might be that a policy of truth-telling is on the whole to one's own advantage; or that it promotes the general welfare; or that it is needed by people who must live together relying on one another.[16]

However there is a problem with Rachels's comments above. His first response is akin to ethical egoism, the second appears to be utilitarianism while the third is reminiscent of contractarianism.[17] For Rachels, strong virtue ethics is flawed because its justification for action-guidance is inadequate. But it is notable that Rachels fails to mention another option, i.e., 'we need the virtues so that we can fare well'; this response – a crude form of neo-Aristotelianism – is clearly not the same as ethical egoism, utilitarianism or contractarianism.

Virtue ethics and the charge of moral relativism

From within a virtue ethics framework, reasons for action will all be related or connected to the virtues and vices. Particular virtues and vices are deemed important in one's life and this depends in part upon one's interests and needs. However, this claim is open to the charge of moral relativism. Critics might argue that no two persons have identical lives and that in many cases, people's interests and needs diverge. It is possible that each person will choose to cultivate only those virtues that will help his/her life to fare well. But this means that different people will cultivate different virtues. Two points spring to mind here. First, there is no guarantee that people will all cultivate the same virtue. Indeed depending on the number of people in question, completely different virtues might be cultivated. For example, out of 100 people 25 cultivate honesty, 25 cultivate patience, another 25 cultivate compassion and the remaining 25 cultivate courage. The second point springs from the first. Each person in this small community believes that the virtue that they cultivate is important to human flourishing; this is, after all, why they chose to cultivate it in the first place. It is alleged that moral relativism reigns because no absolute moral truths are generated by this approach; each person believes that 'their' virtue is the most important one to cultivate. However, while this claim is true as it stands, it fails to accurately represent the precise role of the virtues in morality. The virtues are morally admirable character traits; moral excellences that are good for people to cultivate because they help one's life to go well and tend to benefit others. One can see that in the above example, the cultivation of the four virtues – honesty, patience, compassion and courage – would help their possessor and the other 75 in the community to fare well. But might the 25 people who are honest cause tensions for the remaining 75? Or might those who act courageously cause problems for the others? There is clearly something in this. As it stands, this conception of the virtues might lack sufficient theoretical resources to satisfactorily ground the virtues. This point is picked up again in Chapters 8–11.

The problem of incompleteness – Revisited

The strong virtue ethics approach faces another more general difficulty that is related to the problem of incompleteness. Reasons to do with the virtues and vices help one to know whether to favour or object to an action. Rachels holds that strong virtue ethics must agree with the following claim

> that for any good reason that may be given in favor of doing an action, there is a corresponding virtue that consists in the disposition to accept and act on that reason.[18]

But Rachels thinks this is untrue. For example, suppose one has to decide how to distribute scarce medical resources. One might decide that it is best to do that which will maximize the benefit for the greatest number of people. Rachels asks: 'Is there a virtue that matches this disposition?' He is sceptical that there is and believes that if there is, it should be called 'acting like a utilitarian'. However, this example is quite crude. First, according to obligation-based ethics, the allocation of scarce medical resources will be carried out from the principle of distributive justice. From a virtue ethics perspective, the legislator will be just, act justly and will be fair when allocating the resources. While this will be far from straightforward, acting justly should help to eliminate unjust and partial actions. Considerable action-guidance can be derived from the virtue and vice terms of 'just', 'fair' and 'unfair'. Clearly the virtues of benevolence, honesty and integrity are also important in making these kinds of decisions. Rachels's example concerning the allocation of resources is perhaps too simplistic to be really helpful. Many sources of data will be first identified including epidemiological data on the incidence of AIDS, and data on the incidence of other diseases, for example, coronary heart disease. The allowable expenditure will be identified and a just percentage of the expenditure will be allocated to help those with AIDS, and a just percentage allocated to help those with coronary heart disease and so on. Of course it is not as simple as Rachels or I make out. Many other criteria will be taken into account. However, acting justly and not acting dishonestly in tandem with self-reflection will surely help to prevent injustice.

Conflicts between virtues

It was noted in Chapter 3 that a common objection to the virtue-based approach to morality was conflicts between virtues. Rachels[19] identifies the 'conflict of the virtues' as a serious problem for virtue ethics. How is one meant to resolve situations where two or more virtues have been identified as important? Can the virtues be ranked? For instance, is honesty in a given situation more important than justice? Rachels says:

> Suppose you must choose between A and B, when it would be dishonest but kind to do A, and honest but unkind to do B.[20]

There are moral reasons for and against both telling the truth (and acting unkindly) and withholding information (and acting kindly). Since both kindness and honesty are virtues, it is unclear what one should do. But at the end of the day one must do something. The pronouncement 'act virtuously' clearly fails to help. This is where the idea of ranking the virtues might come in. But can this be done? Rachels fails to provide his response to this question. In response it is not true to say that because honesty and kindness are both virtues, someone will therefore have no idea what to do. As already noted, we need to think deeply about the meaning of each virtue and we need to think hard about what honest and kind persons are like, for example, what characteristically would honest and kind persons do? What behaviours does one expect from honest and kind persons? And what acts would honest and kind persons carry out? Particular circumstances and details will need to be examined and such details will help to shed some light on which virtue is thought more important in a given situation. An example might help. Sally has bought a new dress for a party later that evening. She asks her husband, Tim, what he thinks of it. Tim hates the dress but says that it is lovely. He believes that being honest would be unkind to his wife. He therefore decides to spare her feelings and is instead dishonest believing that this is a kind thing to do. Accounts of honesty as a virtue are very demanding. For example, Hursthouse provides an account of honesty in which she states that the honest person would never lie (tell an untruth), would avoid situations where lying was a possibility, would seek out situations where the truth could be told and would not wish to make friends with people considered dishonest. This interpretation of what it means to be an honest person will not be easy for many people to comply with, but such compliance is necessary in order to be called an honest person (one will also need to think about the meaning of kindness). On this account, Tim was deceiving Sally by intentionally telling her an untruth; in this sense, he was not being honest to her. If he had told the truth, this would have been an act of honesty. Further, he believed that the truth would upset Sally but he failed to give her an opportunity to react to the truth. Sally might have been prepared for the truth. If Tim had not liked the dress, then she might have decided to try on another. Sally bought the dress for a really special occasion (a party) and she wanted to look her best. She now believes that the dress looks good on her partly because of Tim's dishonesty (I say 'partly' because Sally thinks it looks good too and might have bought it irrespective of Tim's views). According to some of Sally's friends, the dress does look good; perhaps Tim's taste in fashion is conservative. At the party, Sally overhears several nasty remarks about her 'dreadful' dress and returns home early in tears. Because Tim is upset at seeing his wife in such a distressed state, he admits that he did not really like the dress. Sally feels annoyed and upset because Tim was dishonest, even though she appreciates his good intentions. Tim regrets his actions and feels upset that he was not honest with his wife. Another point that I think needs making here is that both kindness and honesty are moral virtues. As such, these traits are examples of moral excellences, morally good traits of character that should be praised and admired. Acting from the virtue of kindness and acting from the virtue of honesty are *both* examples of acting *well*. Tim exercised judgement and decided that he should act kindly, but dishonestly. Acting dishonestly is a vice and as such it is an example of acting badly. But I need to stress something here and that is the use of judgement. This is not to be taken lightly. Obligation-based moral theories, for example, the many moral obligations, rules and principles of deontology and the one rule of act-consequentialism, argue that there is no need for people to use judgement in making moral decisions. Instead, one need only abide by the rules, and the morally right course of action will be revealed. Virtue ethics makes exercising judgement fundamentally important to morality and to the aim of persons faring well. Tim took into account lots of information including knowledge of his wife, what sort of person Sally is, which traits she admires in others, previous experiences and perhaps discussions that the couple had had in the past about similar situations. Based on all of these things (and more), Tim made a judgement. The motive and reason for his decision was kindness, therefore his motive was morally good. (I examine the notion of making moral judgements in Chapter 8.) Furthermore, as noted in Chapter 3 obligation-based ethicists are not immune from the conflicts problem. Often a ranking of obligations will need to occur, which is far from satisfactory. Deontology could be charged with failing to resolve conflicts between moral obligations, rules and principles. Things fare better, in this sense, for act-utiltiarians since they have only one rule: 'maximise utility'. But there are many deontological rules that take one of several forms. For example, the rules taught as children by one's parents such as 'Don't lie', 'Tell the truth' and 'Be kind to your elders', Ross's[21] *prima facie* obligations and moral rules proposed in medical ethics by Gert et al.[22]

Can one display a virtue in performing a bad or evil deed?

Both Aristotle and Plato were troubled by this question, and Foot and Benn have also addressed this question. As examples, Benn gives the courage of a terrorist in planting bombs that might kill or injure innocent people and the kindness demonstrated by the 'Robin Hood' thief who steals from the rich to give to the poor. Is the terrorist courageous? Does he not display courage in planting bombs knowing that he could be killed or seriously injured if one exploded? Is the thief really kind or benevolent? He does appear to show some sympathy for the plight of the poor. Benn thinks that one's character is composed of both virtuous and vicious traits. But this is not the problem. His interest instead is in 'whether a particular benevolent act can also be unjust, or a courageous act also cruel?'[23] Benn says:

> if we also allow that the more heedless of human suffering the terrorist is, the more courage he shows, we are implying that if he becomes more compassionate he also becomes less courageous.[24]

This opens the way to call any decrease in his courage, a deficiency. Likewise, let us accept that it is better to be 'perfectly benevolent' than just 'moderately benevolent' Further, accept that one who steals in order to help the poor displays a greater degree of benevolence than someone who refrains from stealing. A troubling implication arises because it appears that one ought to admire those who steal or kill. One response comes from Hursthouse. She believes that a virtue such as courage in a desperado would enable them to carry out 'far more wicked things than they would be able to do if they were timid'.[25] She claims that one arrives at a bizarre thought: that the virtues, which help a person to be morally good, to fare well in life, might end up in fact making a person do morally bad deeds. However, Hursthouse thinks that the desperado is daring rather than courageous. I concur with Hursthouse. In carrying out bad deeds, for example, stealing, a person acts from the vices of dishonesty and injustice. The motive of the Robin Hood thief is not virtuous because in stealing, he does not act well and those people whom he steals from will also not fare well. If I wanted to be sympathetic, I would suggest that this thief was acting like a utilitarian because he was redistributing wealth to maximize the good. Furthermore, the degree of benevolence one develops is not directly proportional to the amount of happiness one creates. For instance, one could be a really kind altruistic person, but fail to create substantial happiness for others; indeed 'happiness' is such an arbitrary subjective term that it becomes almost meaningless. One could be a cruel person and yet make others happy by harming their enemies. Assuming, as Benn does, that it is generally better to create more, rather than less, happiness, this does not licence others to steal or cheat. From a deontological perspective, it is morally wrong to steal because it breaks the moral rule 'one must not steal'. But, from the virtue ethics perspective, stealing is an example of acting badly because it is unjust and dishonest. Thieves can live good lives but not *morally* good lives.

One of the pivotal questions surrounding this debate is: 'Are the ends of human activity good or evil?' Can someone for instance a Nazi soldier show courage when he is fighting for an evil cause? Does courage operate in this case as a virtue? Geach responds to this in no uncertain terms:

> Courage in an unworthy cause is no virtue; still less is courage in an evil cause. Indeed, I prefer not to call this nonvirtuous facing of danger 'courage'.[26]

This makes sense because one does not wish to praise the Nazi soldier for what he does. However, he risks his life and acts in the face of danger. There is undoubtedly something about his actions that suggests that it would be inaccurate not to refer to him as courageous. Rachels attempts to overcome this problem by saying:

> Perhaps we should just say that he displays two qualities of character, one that is admirable (steadfastness in facing danger) and one that is not (a willingness to defend a particular regime). He is courageous all right, and courage is an admirable thing; but because his courage is displayed in an evil cause, his behaviour is *on the whole* wicked.[27]

However, this assumes that the soldier knew at the time that his cause was evil. But in truth how much freedom did a typical Nazi soldier have to refuse to fight? It was expected and obligatory for him to defend his country and most probably, he would have been shot if he had refused to fight; so it might be said that he had no real choice. Irrespective of this, the above quote makes an arbitrary decision about what counts as 'courageous' behaviour. This appears to turn on the perceived goodness or badness of the activity in question. There is a sense in which courage *for any soldier* is clearly a virtue needed in order to survive, protect comrades and fare well. Furthermore, Rachels's response is unconvincing because in my view the notion of 'on the whole behaviour' and the exercise of specific virtues, tends to make an unhappy combination. Foot provides a more convincing response to this problem. She thinks it is wrong (or at least something about this is wrong) when people who have demonstrated apparent virtue, but for a bad or evil end, are praised; an example being the 'courageous' terrorist considered earlier. It remains difficult, however, to say categorically that the terrorist was not in some way courageous – remember he could be killed or seriously injured in the course of planting the bombs. It does appear that the courage shown in trying to achieve good or noble ends is identical to the courage shown by the terrorist in trying to achieve bad or evil ends. The fact that one person decides to achieve bad or evil ends might itself be a sign of a flawed character, a deficiency in virtue. But the deficient virtue is clearly not courage. If one denies that the terrorist shows courage, then one is defining courage arbitrarily to suit one's values. So if one approves of the ends, one might use the word 'courage', whereas when one disapproves of the ends in question another more derogatory term might be used. This usage is termed 'persuasive definition'. According to Benn a good example is the difference between calling a terrorist a 'freedom fighter' or simply a 'terrorist'. Even though the nature of what they do is the same, those who approve of the terrorist's ends will call him a freedom fighter while those who disapprove will call him a terrorist. Foot claims that when courage and benevolence are both displayed in the pursuit of bad or evil ends, '*they do not operate as virtues* in these cases'.[28]

The above point requires further explanation. The foundation for this thought is the idea that 'things do not always operate according to their natures'.[29] Courage, by its nature, is a virtue. In the example of the terrorist, however, it does not operate according to its nature. Other examples given by Benn are prudence and industriousness.[30] Both these operate by their nature as virtues. However, prudence does not operate as a virtue 'in people who are so obsessed with danger that they never take even rational risks'[31] while industriousness does not function as a virtue 'in people who neglect their families to advance their careers'.[32] Despite the earlier claim that one needs the virtues to fare well and lead morally good lives, it seems that there will be times when these traits do not function as virtues because they do not operate according to their natures.

Virtue ethics: Supplementary or strong?

Rachels concludes that a supplementary form of virtue ethics should be adopted because he finds a strong version unconvincing.[33] As noted, however, he has not been able to respond to Hursthouse's v-rules thesis. Rachels is uncertain whether a combined theory could do justice to both the notions of 'right action' and 'virtuous character'. Will one notion be sacrificed to some degree by overemphasizing the other? He thinks that this is highly possible. According to such an overall theory, he suggests that the principal value might be human welfare. It follows then that a major objective will be for all humans to lead satisfying and happy lives. Furthermore, he thinks one needs to consider:

> What sorts of actions and social policies would contribute to this goal *and* the question of which qualities of character are needed to create and sustain individual lives.[34]

According to this combined theory, the nature of virtue 'could profitably be conducted from within the perspective that such a larger view would provide'[35]. In Rachels's view, it would be acceptable for each part of the theory – 'right action' and 'virtuous character' – to be adapted and modified a bit here and there; he believes moral truth will be the benefactor. It is doubtful, however, whether a hybrid version like the one proposed by Rachels could work. This is basically because the starting points for deontic and aretaic theories are fundamentally different; modifying or adjusting one notion whether 'right action' or 'virtuous character' would mark the end of a coherent moral theory (this is a major reason why there are few hybrid theories).[36]

Conclusions

I have examined several common objections levelled at virtue ethics. One of the notable charges against virtue ethics is that it fails to come up with rules and thus cannot provide adequate action-guidance. In Chapter 3, however, I noted that thinking deeply about the virtues and vices can result in plenty of action-guidance. In this chapter, I have discussed Hursthouse's v-rules thesis. I believe that these two claims – first, one's ability to gain action-guidance from the virtues and vices and second, the action-guidance derivable from the v-rules – means that a strong action-guiding version of virtue ethics is a plausible option, certainly more plausible than many critics suppose.

7

A Critical Account of Obligation-Based Moral Theories in Nursing Practice

Introduction

I have established the value of the virtues in the nurse–patient helping relationship and I have argued that a strong version of virtue ethics is plausible. In this chapter, I provide a critical account of obligation-based moral theories in the context of contemporary nursing practice. First, I consider reasons why obligation-based theories are popular in nursing. I examine examples of the deontic approach in the nursing literature and I briefly describe three examples of moral decision-making tools. I then examine the 'four principles' approach to bioethics. I close by highlighting several flaws of obligation-based moral theories as utilized in nursing practice. My conclusion is that these theories are incomplete and inadequate for use as a foundational nursing ethics.

Despite the recognition that nurses should cultivate and exercise the moral virtues, obligation-based moral theories, particularly the four principles approach,[1] remain extremely popular and widespread in the nursing ethics literature[2] and nurse education.[3] Their popularity continues despite sustained critiques.[4]

Why are obligation-based moral theories popular in nursing?

At least three quite obvious reasons spring to mind in response to this question. First, obligation-based moral theories are popular in general ethics; it therefore makes sense to suppose that popular theories in general ethics will be utilized in professional ethics. Second, despite the widespread view that patient-centred and holistic nursing care ought to be key objectives of contemporary nursing practice, a biomedical focus remains predominant.[5] The epistemological paradigm that grounds medical/nursing practice and the biomedical model is empiricism. The focus is firmly on clinical decision-making, including understanding the disease process, making diagnoses, identifying clinical needs, delivering effective treatments and evaluating the outcomes of interventions. As we have seen, consequentialism focuses upon the outcomes of actions. It therefore makes sense that nurses (and doctors) have adopted a consequentialist approach to moral reasoning and decision-making; the moral theory of consequentialism is very much in keeping with the epistemology of empiricism. Third, hospitals are large, complex institutions that in order to operate efficiently rely on people following a system of rules and regulations. Such rules are generally utilitarian or at least consequentialist in nature. This reliance upon rules helps to explain why nurses (and doctors) favour rule-based deontological ethics over other alternative moral theories.

Examples of the deontic approach to moral decision-making in the nursing literature

I shall now briefly describe five examples of the obligation-based approach to moral decision-making in the nursing literature. Essentially, the authors all appear to believe that the moral dilemma is resolvable and they invoke moral obligations, rules and principles in order to do so. The authors seem to claim that there is one right or wrong answer to the dilemma; sometimes, the claim is that of the two harms present, one is less harmful or in some sense more beneficial than the other. The possibility that the dilemma could be irresolvable is not mentioned or at least the authors do not make this possibility explicit.

The first example is Kashka and Keyser[6] who examine ethical concerns in relation to informed consent and ECT by utilizing a principle-based approach and case study. The authors define an ethical quandary in terms of conflicts or tensions caused between two ethical principles, for example, beneficence and autonomy. They conclude that an increased emphasis upon ethical principles is needed from nurses. The authors believe that

> nurses must be grounded in the ethical concepts discussed, [and that] knowledge of the specific situation is also necessary to the decision-making process.[7]

The second example is an introductory chapter from a text on ethics in mental health practice. Kentsmith et al.[8] claim that knowledge of philosophy, ethics and ethical thinking will help nurses make 'better', 'clearer' and more justifiable day to day decisions. Ethics is defined as:

> A branch of philosophy that examines right and wrong, what should or should not be done, and the moral justifications for action.[9]

The authors subdivide ethics into axiology – 'the study of values' – and morality, which is further broken down into teleological, deontological, absolutist and relativistic ethical theories. The authors make no mention of the virtues or virtue ethics and do not raise the question of which character traits are needed to be a morally good nurse; this is a notable omission especially given the remark about axiology and the discussion of the nurse–patient relationship earlier in the chapter. Kentsmith et al. claim that nursing is regulated by ethical codes of conduct. They state that ten ethical principles are implicated in ethical practice including 'a responsibility to the client', 'an obligation to act ethically' and 'a respect for the law'.[10]

In the third example, Hopton[11] considers ethical arguments for and against controlling and restraining (C&R) individuals in severe mental distress. He sketches utilitarian and deontological perspectives in relation to the ethical justification of C&R. With the first, the conclusion is:

> Efficient restraint [the force used must be less injurious than the initial aggressive act] will minimise the harm done to both the restrained person and anyone else.[12]

Hopton holds that deontological arguments are of limited use insofar as there is minimal 'agreement concerning how far a mentally distressed person is accountable for his/her actions'.[13] However, it seems to me that the notion of responsibility and accountability for one's actions while noted as an important issue in nursing, applies equally from a consequentialist perspective. Hopton claims that irrespective of one's ethical perspective an obligation exists for nurses to protect innocent others from the violent acts of the mentally distressed. However, Hopton provides no qualification in relation to his discussion of utilitarianism, so I am uncertain whether he means act or rule utilitarianism or indeed whether he thinks this distinction is unimportant. Such lack of detail regarding moral theories in the nursing ethics literature is not uncommon. As Hursthouse[14] claims sometimes 'slogans' are used to describe moral theories. Therefore as a result of the literature being unsophisticated, nurses may fail to develop a substantial understanding of moral theories including their problems and limitations. Furthermore, Hopton does not present a conception of 'harm' that appears to be central to his discussion. Am I to assume that Hopton believes that emotional suffering is a component of 'harm'? Or is he only referring to physical injury? Surprisingly, there is no explicit mention of one's 'right to psychiatric treatment' and more importantly one's 'rights to refuse treatment'. Finally, although Hopton makes reference to one's need to protect others, no explicit mention is made to obligations to protect innocent others.

In the fourth example, Chodoff[15] distinguishes between and explicates the medical model and the civil liberties approach to the ethical issue of involuntary hospitalization of the mentally ill. He claims that these two different approaches are grounded in respectively, consequentialist and deontological ethics. He claims that issues such as medical necessity versus the notion of 'dangerousness', the role given to rights versus obligations and the justification of medical paternalism depend upon value judgements arising from these different moral perspectives. Because of these issues and because no one has developed a sound method for deriving 'ought' propositions from 'is', there is no certainty about the good and right thing to do in this matter. Of course, in my view these claims – which I concur with – represent some of the serious flaws in obligation-based moral theories that were discussed in Chapter 4 and as such, these criticisms serve as good reasons why alternative moral theories such as virtue ethics should be examined. Chodoff discusses utilitarian versus deontological approaches to ethics. He defines utilitarians as those who

> believe that the morality of an act is determined by the extent to which that act serves the good of individuals or the society.[16]

Whereas, deontologists

> maintain that whether an act has good consequences should not be the only factor determining its rightness or wrongness.[17]

Chodoff claims that the sole criterion for right action besides the 'good' may lie in other intuited principles such as fairness, liberty and justice. The two moral approaches of utilitarianism and deontology are then applied to the ethics of involuntary hospitalization. Chodoff writes:

> The doctors who embrace the medical model are following a utilitarian ideal. For them the removal or diminishing of the barriers that

mental illness imposes on the healthy functioning of their patients is the right thing to do. It justifies temporary deprivation of physical liberty.[18]

However, the civil libertarians see things differently; as Chodoff claims 'they are more concerned with the coercive aspects and with the loss of liberty'. For these thinkers, liberty as a value 'trumps'[19] other values. Chodoff believes that psychiatrists should neither take too lightly the decision to involuntarily commit, nor place extreme emphasis upon the notion of physical liberty. Chodoff provides an adequate definition of utilitarianism, although it is uncertain whether this is meant to encapsulate the doctrines of classical, act or rule utilitarianism. No mention is given to direct or indirect forms of utilitarianism, neither is there further discussion of Chodoff's interpretation of the 'good'. It is also a bit amiss that he fails to discuss the notion of a person's 'interests' as this is fundamental to an adequate picture of utilitarianism. For example, he does not mention that strict classical utilitarians hold that everyone's interests ought to be treat equally and impartially, i.e., no special relationships such as doctor–patient are acknowledged. Chodoff briefly mentions 'obligations' in the article. However, he fails to discuss this or the 'duty of care' further. Despite these minor criticisms, Chodoff's article deserves praise because it at least facilitates a discussion of morality and moral issues rather than focusing on legal obligations and rights. There are occasions when so-called moral or ethical debates actually turn out to be discussions about the law, legal rights and legal obligations. This is the case across all nursing specialities, but it is particularly true regarding mental health nursing where the two disciplines of ethics and law tend to merge together and the boundaries can become blurred.

In the final example, Brown discusses 'a number of key ethical issues with regard to drug treatment'.[20] First, he considers the risks and benefits of drug treatment; this includes a brief section on the boundaries of mental illness. Second, the doctor–patient relationship and the notion of informed consent are scrutinized. Next, he discusses the patient's moral and legal rights with regard to drug treatment and finally, Brown briefly examines the issues of drug costs and social justice. It is notable that Brown does not propose a specific moral argument; instead he reviews ideas concerning patient's rights although he does not philosophize on these.

Three points need noting regarding this review of the deontic literature in nursing practice. First, many other articles are synonymous in their approach to the five described.[21] Second, in describing traditional accounts of obligation-based moral theories the authors fail to regard the virtues as important to the ends of being a morally good nurse.[22] And third, subsequent literature searches conducted in 2002–2005 yielded similar findings; however, to be accurate several articles on the place of virtue ethics in nursing have been published within the past two years.[23]

Moral decision-making tools

As noted in Chapter 4, one of the aims of the obligation-based approach to moral decision-making in general ethics is to resolve moral dilemmas.[24] In an attempt to facilitate the resolution of moral dilemmas, several authors have proposed decision-making tools. In briefly describing three such tools, I aim to illustrate some of the assumptions made by the obligation-based approach to moral decision-making.

In the first example, Kentsmith et al. claim that using 'systematic problem solving tools' can enhance 'the analysis of ethical dilemmas'.[25] Their approach consists of the following six 'stages': determine the facts, analyse the ethical aspects, outline the options, make a decision, take action and evaluate the decision. For novice nurses in particular, moral decision-making tools or 'models' can help to clarify some of the moral issues. However, these 'stages' are conceptual tools that require application by nurses who need to think carefully and ask questions about a wide range of moral and clinical issues. The second example is Ericksen's theoretical framework model, which consists of five areas of knowledge: knowledge of oneself and one's values; knowledge of the situation; knowledge of the profession's values and standards; knowledge of the law; and knowledge of philosophy. By adopting this framework, it is claimed that it is possible 'to make a decision that will be in the best interests of both nurse and client'.[26] However, the utility of this framework will be determined by several factors including the nurse's breadth and depth of understanding regarding the five areas of knowledge; there is also the difficult philosophical debate regarding the nature and meaning of 'best interests' to consider.[27] The third example is by McAlpine et al.[28] who dissatisfied with current measuring instruments[29] developed the ethical reasoning tool (ERT) to measure nurses' ability regarding ethical reasoning. The ERT measures nurses' unprompted thinking about practice dilemmas rather than asking nurses to rank existing lists of issues. The authors claim that the ERT could be used to evaluate the teaching of ethics modules and to detect deficient areas of students' ethical reasoning. While I believe that it is valuable to gain an empirical understanding of moral reasoning especially if it leads to beneficial changes in the teaching of ethics to nurses, it is unclear what the ERT actually measures. For example, it might measure a nurse's understanding of the question or a nurse's ability to be articulate. None of these moral decision-making tools examines or even refers to a nurse's moral character. Instead these tools place the emphasis on the action itself, but fail to adequately consider the person (nurse) who actually performs the action.

The four principles approach to biomedical ethics

Beauchamp and Childress[30] first proposed the four principles approach to biomedical ethics in 1979 (henceforth, I shall refer to this approach as 'principlism'). Principlism consists of four *prima facie* moral principles, namely, beneficence, non-maleficence, justice and respect for autonomy. Beauchamp and Childress hav e influenced many ethicists and in the UK, thinkers such as Edwards[31] and Gillon[32] advocate principlism. Principlism can be understood as four second-order moral obligations derived from the first-order moral theory of deontology. It is, however, difficult to be more specific because the underlying philosophical foundation appears to derive from what Hursthouse calls 'simple' deontology.[33] The claim that principlism is a coherent moral theory has itself been attacked[34] and while Beauchamp appears to be a deontologist, Childress seems to be a utilitarian. However, there is no doubt that principlism is a highly influential and popular obligation-based approach to moral decision-making. Because principlism is so popular in the literature and in both clinical ethics and nurse education, I shall discuss each principle in more detail.

The principle of non-maleficence

The principle of non-maleficence is essentially concerned with minimizing harms and balancing benefits against harms. For example, a nurse notes that a patient taking lithium is experiencing excessive shakes and this is causing the patient some distress. The nurse consults with the psychiatrist and the dose of lithium is lowered. The patient's symptoms remain controlled, but the shakes cease. In this example, the nurse has acted from the principle of non-maleficence. This principle appears to be morally weightier than the principle of beneficence. Simply put, since it is not always possible to benefit a patient it is considered morally more important to minimize harms. However, I am concerned that traditional accounts of consequentialism and deontology portray the notions of 'benefits' and 'harms' in a myopic sense; or to be more precise, nurses are more likely to conceive these notions in a limited sense, one that is perhaps exclusively focused on physical benefits and harms. Compare this to the virtue-based perspective that as we saw earlier, conceives that the virtue of kindness motivates a wide range of actions, thoughts and feelings. I am not saying that the obligation-based approach precludes a nurse from 'thinking outside of the box', i.e., this approach does not necessarily mean that nurses will think only in terms of physical benefits and harms. However, because the virtue-based approach does not over-focus on the nature or consequences of actions, there is more scope and opportunity for nurses to think of a wider range of actions, thoughts and feelings. Clouser and Gert[35] view the obligation of non-maleficence as unproblematic. However, they prefer to frame it in terms of the moral rules that they espouse, for example, 'don't kill, don't cause pain and don't disable'.[36] According to Clouser and Gert, the obligation of non-maleficence is straightforward because it does not blur the distinction between moral ideals,[37] which concern the prevention of harms and moral rules,[38] which concern the avoidance of harms.

The principle of justice

This principle is often seen solely in terms of distributive justice, for example, how ought scarce medical resources to be allocated?[39] However, retributive justice addresses such important ideas as blame and punishment, and is therefore also important in nursing ethics.[40] According to the principle of justice, nurses should treat patients fairly and impartially irrespective of one's values and beliefs. Patients' individual needs should be identified and taken into account fairly in planning and delivering nursing care. Beauchamp notes that different theories of justice have been proposed. He writes:

> To cite one example, an egalitarian theory of justice implies that if there is a departure from equality in the distribution of health care benefits and burdens, such a departure must serve the common good and enhance the position of those who are least advantaged in society.[41]

As with all principles, the principle of justice can mean different things depending upon which theory of justice is utilized. Clouser and Gert attack this principle because it 'does not even pretend to provide a specific guide to action'.[42] This criticism illustrates a general concern regarding principlism, i.e., that it does not provide a coherent philosophical foundation. As a result one is left without the necessary theoretical ammunition with which to make justifiable moral decisions. For example, on the Beauchamp and Childress account of the principle of justice all that is offered are instructions concerning matters of distribution and recommendations towards the fair allocation of resources. But one of the problems is that one is not given a definite account of any theory of justice. Because of this sort of omission, some critics allege that principlism is 'empty'.[43] Moreover, according to Clouser and Gert, the principle of justice blurs the distinction between moral rules and moral ideals.

The principle of respect for autonomy[44]

Beauchamp describes 'respect for autonomy' as 'the obligation to respect the decision-making capacities of autonomous persons'.[45] It seems to me that this principle represents the core of their approach to biomedical ethics; this now appears to be the predominant moral principle.[46] The Western liberal tradition that emphasizes human freedom, liberty and human rights is one of the reasons why this principle is seen to be so important.[47] Recently, *The Patient's Charter*[48] and the Human Rights Act[49] have increased patients' awareness of moral and legal rights in particular rights to refuse treatments. In contemporary health care ethics, the moral responsibility of nurses appears to be understood

> in terms of the rights of persons-in-care, including autonomy-based rights to truthfulness, confidentiality, privacy, disclosure and consent, as well as welfare rights rooted in claims of justice.[50]

A moral requirement of autonomy-based rights involves allowing others to make their own health care decisions; in other words, to promote personal rule, which needs to be

> free from both controlling interferences by others and from personal limitations that prevent meaningful choice, such as inadequate understanding.[51]

Of course, it is not particularly clear what 'meaningful choice' actually consists in. For example, even if it is agreed that an individual is acting autonomously, it is difficult to know which act truly represents the autonomous nature of the chooser.[52] Childress claims that health care professionals should pursue autonomy for their patients. He believes that autonomy is an end state of health, but he also stresses that one should be aware that 'individuals may autonomously choose not to pursue [autonomy]'.[53] For example, a person might visit his doctor and ask his doctor to 'sort me out'. This person trusts his doctor totally and respects his doctor's expertise, which is why he is willing to allow his doctor to 'do his job', but this patient's choice remains an autonomous one. Gillon defines autonomy as:

> The capacity to think, decide and act on the basis of such thought and decision, freely and independently, and without, as it says in the British passport, let or hindrance.[54]

Gillon makes another crucial point, namely, that one's acts and choices should be voluntary and not hindered or prevented by unwanted interference. At least one general 'component' of autonomy is the notion of self-determination. Others share this view; for example, Kashka and Keyser define autonomy as 'one's right to self govern, to assert individual choice'.[55] This capacity – to think, decide, choose and act for oneself – is considered a good and is widely encouraged. Similarly, 'thinking for oneself' and 'getting by independently' are typically seen in a positive light and people are usually praised for having these qualities. I believe that the meaning of the notion of autonomy is far from clear both in theory and in nursing practice. It is more complex than often realized and involves many strands of thought pertaining to broad and deep areas of human life. Nevertheless, some consensus is reached on a 'minimum conception' of autonomy, for example, allowing competent patients to make their own decisions (even if other people deem their decisions to be bad).

Respect for autonomy

Having sketched a basic conception of autonomy, what might it mean to *respect* someone's autonomous decisions? In response to this question, Downie and Calman suggest that

> to *respect* a person as an autonomous being ... is to take into account in one's conduct that he/she has an autonomous nature, that he/she is self-determining and self-governing or that he/she has desires, feelings and reason.[56]

Precisely *how* can a nurse show respect for a patient's choice? Does a nurse show respect if she asks a patient for his view on having a treatment such as chemotherapy or ECT? Perhaps this is part of the answer but surely showing respect concerns more than *just* asking someone for their view. Is respect shown when a nurse asks a patient for his view *and* listens closely to his reply? Again, I can listen to my wife's views on, for example, the quality of situation comedies on UK TV, but if I proceed to ridicule my wife's views, then my behaviour might upset her; behaving in this manner does not demonstrate respect for my wife's views (although this is perhaps different from disrespecting my wife). Does a nurse respect a patient's choice by telling him openly that she disagrees with his choice? This is certainly an honest thing to do. Respect might be shown if the nurse listened closely to what the patient said and made it clear to him that she valued his view. Indeed, I would suggest that a large part of showing respect to anyone involves communicating well (see the discussion of the nurse–patient relationship in Chapter 2). Finally, is respect shown *if and only if* despite disagreeing with a patient's choice the nurse and multidisciplinary team *accept* the patient's decision? It is clear that showing respect (and disrespect) is a complex notion that requires serious thought.

The principle of beneficence

For centuries, the accepted goal of medicine has been one of medical beneficence, and it remains the case that nurses (doctors and health care professionals) ought to serve this particular end of health care. According to Beauchamp:

> The principle of beneficence expresses an obligation to help others further their important and legitimate interests by preventing and removing harms; no less important is the obligation to weigh and balance possible goods against the possible harms of an act.[57]

Kashka and Keyser claim that beneficence should be outcome centred. They believe that 'doing good for clients, or acting in their best interests is the primary value [in nursing]'.[58] In their view, beneficence 'involves the perceived duty to "do good", to contribute to the welfare and happiness of others'.[59] In relation to beneficence, Frankena states:

> We ought to do the act or follow the practice or rule that will or probably will bring about the greatest possible balance of good over evil.[60]

One should note that Frankena provides a utilitarian interpretation of beneficence. Other possible conceptions of beneficence include rights-based (libertarian) and virtue-based; the latter views benevolence (including kindness) to be the corresponding virtue to the obligation of beneficence. Irrespective of the philosophical underpinnings, the moral foundation of nursing remains the obligation of beneficence. The motivation for nurses to 'do good' comes from several sources including patients, patients' relatives, the UK's Nursing and Midwifery Council (NMC), society's expectations, one's colleagues and of course one's own moral values. According to this principle, nurses are obliged to benefit patients. Examples of acting from the principle of beneficence are too numerous to list, but include: administering paracetamol to a patient to alleviate a headache; repositioning someone in bed to prevent a pressure sore; administering chemotherapy to kill cancer cells; providing ECT to treat depression; feeding a patient and comforting a patient by listening to his narrative account of illness. Clouser and Gert make the charge that this principle (along with justice and autonomy) makes a serious error. They claim that it blurs the distinction between moral ideals and moral rules. Furthermore, they criticize this principle because it fails 'to distinguish between the preventing (or relieving) of evil and the conferring (or promoting) of goods'.[61] Clouser and Gert argue that to prevent or relieve harm one may be justified in violating certain moral rules, whereas no such justification would be possible when merely conferring benefits.

A major criticism of principlism is that it ignores the role of the virtues in the moral lives of patients and nurses. It was not until the fourth edition of *Principles of Biomedical Ethics* in 1994 that the topic of the virtues and a corresponding virtue ethic was thoughtfully, yet still only partially, debated. In the 2004 edition, the authors have further improved the text by including a substantial chapter on the role of the virtues in biomedicine and an adequate account of virtue ethics as an alternative moral theory.

Criticisms of obligation-based moral theories in nursing

In Chapter 4, I critiqued obligation-based moral theories in general ethics. Some of these criticisms have already been reiterated in this chapter. I shall now summarize seven criticisms of obligation-based moral theories utilized in nursing ethics.

First, obligation-based moral theories, for example, consequentialism and deontology focus, respectively, on the consequences and nature of actions/omissions. According to these theories, nurses are obliged to act in accordance with certain moral obligations, rules and principles. As a result of an over-focus on 'action(s)' and the notion of 'morally *right* (and *wrong*) actions', other morally relevant features such as virtues are ignored and neglected; for example, the moral character of the person (both nurse and patient) is glossed over. Furthermore, other morally important features are typically overlooked, for example, how should the meaning and content of the obligations be applied? Moreover, the role of the emotions in the moral lives of nurses and patients tend not to be appreciated and examined; for example, the issue of how a nurse might *feel* during and after moral dilemmas is not debated. Second, the aims of obligation-based theories include revealing the 'resolution' of moral dilemmas. As highlighted in the literature that was discussed earlier in this chapter and in Chapter 4, there is a danger that an assumption is made that all moral dilemmas and all morally complex situations can always be 'satisfactorily' resolved. My view is that this assumption is false and far too simplistic; in each moral dilemma there will be many different ways of addressing the moral conflicts, but depending on whose interests take priority it is likely that none of the options will be entirely satisfactory. Third, obligation-based moral theories, in particular act-utilitarianism but also forms of deontology, tend to neglect the role of judgement in the moral life of nurses. This is in sharp contrast to the reality of contemporary nursing practice.[62] Also, there is no discussion or examination of the notion of moral wisdom, which is another important consideration concerning how nurses *make* moral judgements. In essence, it seems that the reality of clinical nursing is not acknowledged. Fourth, as noted in Chapter 4, obligation-based theories especially deontology, fail to provide sufficient action-guidance for nurses in order to resolve the myriad of conflicts between obligations that arise daily in nursing practice. Attempts at assigning different moral weights to distinct obligations do not go far enough; nurses are thus left without the necessary conceptual tools in order to clarify complex, multidimensional conflicts. Fifth, the notions and concepts utilized in obligation-based theories are evaluative in nature. As a result it is difficult, if not impossible, to arrive at shared meanings and common understandings of such evaluative notions. For example, the notions of 'harms', 'benefits', 'interests' and 'respect' are all far from simple to fully comprehend. This is not an ideal situation especially for novice nurses who are perhaps left (a) bewildered at the complexity of the discipline of ethics or in my view worse, (b) certain that by simply following a moral obligation a morally correct/right action will be guaranteed. Sixth, typically traditional accounts of obligation-based moral theories tend not to debate the moral education of nurses, for example, how and why should nurses be taught to be morally good nurses? Finally, it seems to me that obligation-based moral theories cohere tightly with the biomedical model. I have mentioned how the empirical paradigm of medicine emphasizes certain features of clinical practice, for example, clinical outcomes. I have suggested that one of the reasons why consequentialism is a popular theory is because of its focus on the consequences of actions and omissions. However, contemporary nursing is trying to move away from 'doing tasks' and 'achieving good results', and instead it is aiming to promote and deliver patient-centred and holistic nursing care. If nurses only utilize obligation-based moral theories, then there is a danger that the aims and objectives of these theories will conflict with and perhaps oppose the objectives of contemporary nursing. Rather than the relational and narrative perspective taken by virtue ethics, I view obligation-based ethics as detached theories because their focus is not on the person – the patient, nurse and others – but the act itself.

Conclusions

Adopting an obligation-based moral approach in nursing practice inevitably means that nurses are compelled to abide by certain moral obligations, for example, beneficence. This approach focuses on the nature and consequences of actions, especially the idea of right and wrong actions. The Right – i.e., aiming to do the right actions – is seen as prior to the Good – i.e., being a morally good nurse. The emphasis is on *right* (correct) actions instead of morally *good* nurses, good moral character and morally good actions. Note that 'the' morally right action/decision is not necessarily equivalent to a morally good deed (this important idea was discussed in Chapter 4).

One of the major problems with moral obligations is that they are social constructs, which are conceived by people to help explain the world; in this case morality and ethics. Social constructs such as obligations are external to the person; therefore these features might not seamlessly integrate with the kind of person (nurse) one is. In other words, obligations that instruct nurses to act in particular ways might not represent the natural character of the nurse. So, for example, a cruel nurse can still benefit a patient, perhaps by giving him paracetamol for a headache. It is quite clear that this act – giving paracetamol – has a beneficent effect. However, it is less clear what the nurse's motive is. Perhaps she would respond by saying that she acted from the duty of beneficence. But it has been noted (in Chapters 3 and 5) that something of value is missing from actions that are not performed from the virtues. Moreover, if this nurse acts according to the obligation-based approach then it is possible that she will not adequately consider *kind thoughts* and *feelings*; and she might not reflect on how these sorts of morally relevant features can have a positive impact on the lives of patients. Furthermore, from my experience of teaching ethics to both students and qualified nurses it appears that there is some blurring between moral and legal obligations, responsibilities and rights. Quite understandably perhaps, instead of nurses' practice being guided by moral virtues or moral obligations, their practice is according to at least some studies motivated by legal obligations and rights.[63]

Traditional accounts of obligation-based moral theories hold that nurses who do not abide by moral/professional obligations have in some sense failed their 'professional' status as nurses and could – depending on the particulars – be held blameworthy for their actions/omissions. For example, an admirable nurse with an unblemished career ends up in dispute with the NMC because she was deemed to contravene or breach a specific professional rule. Perhaps in the circumstances the precise rule was one that the nurse felt was harsh and inflexible. Perhaps she acted well to help the patient. However, despite acting from the virtue of, for example, kindness or honesty the nurse is suspended and investigated by the NMC. It was thought that her kindness breached a professional rule set forth by the NMC in its Code of Conduct.[64] But does one episode of 'rule-breaking' warrant the premature end of a clinically and morally excellent nurse's career? Codes of conduct are clearly important for the protection of the public from clinically incompetent and morally corrupt or bad nurses. If nurses wish to fare well in a professional sense, then they need to abide by, or at least not contravene, the code of conduct. However, this does not mean that codes of conduct[65] in general and the NMC code in particular are without their problems. The NMC code is both deontological and consequentialist in content and focuses on patients' interests, outcomes and benefits. It fails, however, to provide conceptual adequacy. Furthermore, despite the contemporary emphasis on effective, high-quality care there is a definite failure – a lost opportunity – to identify and examine the important role played by moral virtues in the work of nurses and the impact of the virtues in providing morally excellent care.

In this chapter I have summarized several common criticisms of obligation-based moral theories in nursing ethics. Four notable flaws of these theories are: (1) their neglect of the moral character of nurses and patients; (2) their overfocus on the nature and consequences of actions; (3) their ignorance of the crucial role played by emotion in the moral lives of patients and nurses; and (4) the incompatibility of obligation-based moral theories with the current emphasis upon and desire to promote patient centered and holistic nursing care. Because of these (and other) flaws, obligation-based moral theories are incomplete and inadequate as a nursing ethics. In the next chapter, I apply the virtue-based approach to morality to contemporary nursing practice.

8
Virtue-Based Moral Decision-Making in Nursing Practice

Introduction

I shall begin this chapter by summarizing several points made in Chapter 2. First, illness causes people to feel certain emotions, for example vulnerability, helplessness and powerlessness, and these feelings can be intensified through the process of hospitalization. Second, patients depend on nurses for help to meet their interests and needs and this is effectively achieved by means of the helping or therapeutic nurse–patient relationship. Third, nurses' roles are multifaceted and difficult to generalize, however it is widely agreed that the development and sustenance of a helping nurse–patent relationship is a vital role of the nurse. Fourth, in essence nurses help to ensure that patients survive and fare well during illness and strive hard to enable their recovery from illness; or when dealing with terminally ill patients, nurses help to ensure patients have good deaths.[1] Fifth, while illness forms only one aspect of a patient's life nurses can view the patient's illness in the form of a narrative. To understand the narrative, a nurse needs to converse with the patient and desire to listen to the patient's lived experience of illness. This approach is in sharp contrast with the medical model. Sixth, according to samples of patients and patients' relatives, being a 'good' nurse and providing 'high-' quality care includes such issues and themes as nurses spending time with patients, nurses getting to know patients and nurses listening to patients. Again according to samples of patients and patients' relatives, the helping nurse–patient relationship is valued as highly as or more highly than other clinical interventions. Empirical evidence from nurses suggests that being a 'good' nurse requires both practical abilities and moral qualities; the latter include demonstrating honesty, compassion and trustworthiness.

In earlier chapters, I presented my conception of a moral virtue and I examined supplementary and strong versions of virtue ethics arguing that the latter are plausible and defensible. Having critiqued obligation-based moral theories in general ethics, in the previous chapter I argued that such theories are inadequate as a nursing ethics. In this chapter I shall focus on one of the merits of the virtue-based approach to morality and apply it to nursing. This is the crucial role played by judgement and moral wisdom in the moral lives of persons. I hope to demonstrate how nurses can use judgement, moral wisdom and the virtues to make morally good decisions. As an example, I consider the virtue of compassion. I refer to the exercise of the virtues and the use of judgement and moral wisdom as the virtue-based approach to morality or moral decision-making. Besides the use of judgement and moral wisdom, I examine other merits of the virtue-based approach. Then, I discuss some common problems of the virtue-based approach in particular the 'conflicts between virtues' problem that I highlighted in Chapters 3 and 5. I end the chapter by arguing that the virtue-based approach is a viable and plausible rival to the traditional obligation-based moral theories of utilitarianism and deontology.

Judgement and moral wisdom

Judgement

In Chapter 4, Hursthouse[2] examined the SCT. There were two distinct parts to this thesis: (a) moral obligations, rules and principles amount to a decision procedure to determine the *right action* in *any* particular case and (b) this decision procedure needs to be stated in terms so that a non-virtuous person could understand and apply it correctly. Act-utilitarianism states that the morally right course of action will be revealed through application of its single rule 'maximize best consequences'. However, as noted in Chapters 4 and 5 one of the criticisms of obligation-based theories is that their portrayal of the moral life and moral experiences is too simplistic and straightforward than it really is. If we look again at the SCT above, the italicized words clearly show that the focus is on telling people what the 'right action' is and this is grounded in the belief that it is always possible to determine what the right action will be irrespective of the circumstances. I am not going to repeat all of the objections levelled at obligation-based moral theories that were discussed in Chapters 4 and 7. But I wish to focus for a moment on the phrase 'morally relevant features' that frequently appears in the ethics literature. I believe that these features include the following concepts or qualities: (1) the consequences or outcomes of acts and omissions, (2) duty-based intentions and motives, (3) the nature, content and application of moral obligations, rules and principles, (4) rights-based reasons, (5) moral virtues including virtue-based intentions and motives, (6) people's interests, needs and values, (7) intuitions and (8) religious beliefs. In nursing practice, I believe that other issues such as past experiences and clinical knowledge are also relevant.[3] One can see that obligation-based theories fail to discuss several important and necessary features of the moral life. These theories at least in their traditional forms as discussed in Chapter 4 – tend to over focus on (1)–(3); or perhaps if the theory is deontological, then there might be room to accommodate (4). Traditional accounts of obligation-based moral theories seem to claim that other morally important features such as the moral character of persons are unimportant in providing an adequate account of morality, moral decision-making and the moral lives of persons.

But of course something is missing from the above list. What do people use to make decisions and choices? My response is simple: judgement. Note what I said above about act-utilitarianism and the application of its single rule. Take an example such as the morality of breaking a promise. It might well be that act-utilitarianism, deontology and virtue ethics agree that the right thing to do is that that minimizes suffering. But for virtue ethics the process of getting to this resolution is not as simple as it is for the other two theories. Virtue ethics uses judgement to ask questions such as was this the sort of promise that should never have been made? Should it be broken? What might some of the effects be if the promise is broken? One can see that questions can be framed in terms of the promise and the consequences of breaking it. Of course, questions should also address the people involved, for example, what does the breaking of this promise say about the character of the person who breaks it? If it was a silly extravagant promise, what does this say about the person who made it? Discussing the notion of 'consequences' does not present problems for virtue ethicists; I would suggest that despite their moral allegiance all ethicists realize that the notion of consequences/outcomes *is* important in morality. But the acknowledgement that consequences are important in morality is very different from constructing a moral theory *based* on the notion of consequences particularly when such a theory excludes other equally important moral features.[4] I believe that part (a) of Hursthouse's SCT is a fair representation of the aim of obligation-based moral theories. Turning to deontology for a moment, common moral rules such as 'do not lie' are undoubtedly important in morality and especially in educating the young to 'do the right thing'. Virtue ethics talks about the virtue of honesty and the vice of dishonesty; its pivotal objective is to educate the young to be good persons. It is clear that the moral rule 'do not lie' and the virtue of honesty are related. Virtue ethics does not need to reject deontology's rules. However, Hursthouse[5] believes that instead of merely teaching children about rules and the need to abide by such rules, it is crucial that children are taught to love and prize the truth by teaching the virtue of honesty. I agree with this claim. It seems to me that there are several differences between the two approaches, which have been examined in Chapters 3–7 and two differences are worth reiterating here. First, it comes back to moral motives: should someone tell the truth in a particular case because he has been taught that he must abide by certain rules such as 'never lie'? Or should one tell the truth because one understands that it is good to be honest, that morally speaking honesty is a virtue and people benefit from it, and that morally speaking, dishonesty is an example of acting badly? Second, it should be clear by now that morality is not *just* about actions and actors; thus an account of right action is just one requirement of an adequate moral theory. Virtue ethics emphasizes the role of moral character, for example, it asks what kind of person should I be? Virtue ethics recognizes that besides the consequences and nature of acts/omissions, thoughts and feelings are also morally important phenomena.

I believe that act and rule consequentialism are incomplete and inadequate moral theories. I have given my reasons in Chapters 4 and 7, and one or two have been briefly noted above. I also have serious objections against deontology. However, from a virtue ethics perspective deontology's rules tend to be reasonable; they make sense and I can see how useful they are in moral education. I am therefore reluctant to cast all of deontology's rules aside without further reflection. If people are to find deontology's moral rules helpful and acceptable, there are at least four points that I would like addressed. First, rules should be clearly articulated and framed to allow 'ordinary' people (i.e., non-philosophers) to understand them. Second, such rules need to be specific enough to provide relevant action-guidance, but should also be flexible enough to apply them with success in different circumstances. Third, justification for the rules should be clearly set forth, explaining the rule's origin and why it is important. Situations involving conflicts between rules are unavoidable. Thus, fourth, explicit acknowledgement of such conflicts should be evident and a suitable 'method' of resolving such conflicts should be clearly explicated. However, deontological theories remain incomplete and inadequate (as discussed in Chapter 4). Moral rules, obligations and principles are not sufficient in morality. One major point that appears to receive minimal attention by deontologists is that moral rules are not somehow magically applied. Instead, people actually determine how the rules are applied. For example, nurses apply the rules, obligations and principles of deontology (and the rule of act-consequentialism). Two nurses might apply a specific rule for instance 'do not breach confidential information' in different ways. One may reveal a piece of information that the other nurse would not. Or two nurses acting from the obligation of beneficence[6] might act in distinct ways. This is partly because the nature of obligation-based concepts is evaluative. For instance, taking two common moral rules as examples, what might it mean to (a) 'promote the patients' *interests*' and (b) 'do no *harm* to the patient'? Besides the evaluative nature of moral rules, obligations and principles, another necessary consideration regarding the different ways that a nurse can act is the moral character of the nurse applying the rule. This is why an examination of the virtues and vices and a corresponding virtue ethics is so important. The need for a nurse to exercise judgement is important because (as noted above) moral rules are evaluative and thus can be conceived and interpreted in different ways. Furthermore, the range of morally relevant features (as listed on p. 127) is broad. The NMC code of conduct also aims to provide nurses with action-guidance; it is clearly deontological in content, however, because it talks about 'interests' and 'outcomes' it also espouses a crude form of consequentialism. I say 'crude' because the code lacks philosophical analysis and argumentation. Judgement is utilized in deliberating on all of the possible morally relevant features of situations; for instance, nurses need to ask questions about their importance in a given situation. They also need to evaluate their meaning and utility and reflect on possible difficulties and limitations with each one.

Moral wisdom

Virtue ethics states that persons should use the virtues and judgement to make morally good decisions. Hursthouse goes further and recognizes the notion known as 'moral wisdom'. For her, this complex phenomenon contains three components: moral perception, moral sensitivity and moral imagination. I am reluctant to claim that these components are sufficient for moral wisdom, but they are clearly involved and worthy of further examination.

Moral perception

Several thinkers have drawn attention to the role of emotion in moral thinking including moral perception and sensitivity.[7] For example, Oakley believes that emotion is a necessary feature of moral perception and that without it, moral perception is diminished. According to Aristotle (see Chapter 5), perception allows people to see and understand specific facts, circumstances and details of situations that enable one to exercise a virtue to the right degree. Lutzen and Nordin[8] conducted a grounded theory study involving 14 psychiatric nurses, each with a minimum of five years post-registration experience in mental health nursing. The broad aim of the study was to reveal additional dimensions of moral decision-making. Interviews were carried out with each nurse; one question was asked:

> Can you tell me about a situation in which you had to make a decision concerning patient care but were unsure what was right or wrong.[9]

The method of constant comparative analysis revealed the core concept: structuring moral meaning. There were three interrelated properties to the core concept: perceiving, knowing and judging. According to the authors, 'perceiving'

> in relationship to moral conflicts is the capacity in which the nurse discerns meaning in her observations in order to comprehend the reality of the situation.[10]

Perception will be understood according to Lutzen and Nordin's conception above. Simply put, it is one's capacity to see and provide meaning in observations and experiences. The range of observations and experiences that nurses can perceive is vast. I see no point in even attempting to provide a list of such observations and experiences. Some examples of these are given in this book. If I presented such a list, it would be a form of crude reductionism: richly textured, complex and multilayered personal experiences described in a few short sentences. One of the key points is that nursing is saturated with morally and emotionally complex situations. So much happens at an intrapersonal and interpersonal level that it is difficult for nurses to perceive well. There will be occasions when specific information is not perceived. Several factors can affect one's ability to perceive. One's knowledge base is clearly important including clinical knowledge of illness. If a nurse understands aspects of an illness then thoughts will be triggered that will enable her to search for specific signs, or questions will be asked that seek to identify certain possible symptoms. Two other factors that might affect the quality of perception are time and the emotional well-being of the nurse. In brief, if there is insufficient time for a nurse to deliver all interventions, then less time might be spent in direct contact with patients; a nurse might need to work at a faster pace so that she can manage to meet patients' needs. This situation can be intensified if a nurse is emotionally and physically tired. Moral perception concerns one's ability to see, discern meaning and understand the wide range of morally relevant features that might be involved in particular interactions. Previous actions need to be reflected on and nurses should reflect on the patient's illness; in part these activities will promote one's ability to perceive and evaluate situations. From the examination of consequentialist and deontological moral theories in Chapters 4 and 7, it seems to me that neither of these theories emphasizes moral perception. Indeed the phenomenon of moral wisdom tends to be ignored by traditional obligation-based moral theorists; however, several contemporary nurse ethicists realize the importance of this phenomenon.[11] It is important to note that obligation-based moral theorists are not precluded from examining moral wisdom including moral perception. However, the moral rules espoused by deontology and the one rule of act-consequentialism – 'maximize best consequences' – hold that judgement is unnecessary in determining the morally right action.

Is it possible to shed more light on the meaning of 'judging'? When I judge a song, for example, I listen to it. I think about its composition, I consider how the music and lyrics work together and I think about the song's emotional effect on me. Am I moved by it? What do I think about when I listen to it? How do I feel when I listen to it? I might compare one song with another written by the same artist and I will think about similarities and differences. If a friend asks me for a judgement on a particular song, then I will give him my opinion. In this way, my judgement is a conscious decision based on a process of reasoning and reflection. When I make judgements, I am making choices. If the object of a judgement is aesthetic, for example, music, then such a judgement is based on certain personal values and beliefs. For instance, while listening to a song, I tend to prefer to listen to the music rather than the lyrics, but another person might focus on the lyrics. This is an example of a value judgement. There is a sense in which all judgements are based on values; thus judgements, conceived as decisions and choices, are subjective and personal. In the Lutzen and Nordin[12] study, the process of judging was found to involve two aspects referred to as valuing and idealizing. According to the authors, these aspects 'refer to the dialectical components, personal values and professional ideals, in judging alternatives'.[13] This claim relates to the conflicts experienced by nurses between, on the one hand, the rules laid down by institutions such as hospitals and rules proposed in professional codes of conduct and, on the other hand, one's own value and belief systems. Several empirical studies suggest that nurses use intuition and instincts in making moral decisions in nursing practice. For example, Lutzen and Nordin[14] found that nurses relied heavily upon intuition and 'feelings' for moral perception rather than moral theories such as principle-based ethics.[15] One conclusion drawn from this study 'indicates that moral decision making within the nurse–patient relationship is not always deduced from rational thinking or principles'.[16] Moreover, rather than moral principles or codes of conduct nurses focus on responses towards patients and take different contexts into account regarding the nurse–patient relationship in defining their own choices and decisions.[17] Furthermore, in terms of moral perception, nurses see, understand and communicate morally complex situations using the language of the virtues and vices, for example, 'fair', 'care', 'well' and 'honest'.[18] Experiential evidence derived from almost 20 years of clinical experience leads me to concur with these empirical studies. For some nurses, formal moral theory does not appear to be useful. Indeed my personal experience is that even with substantial knowledge of moral theory and health care ethics, reflecting on my clinical career I would conclude that my moral decision-making was grounded in intuition and emotions/feelings towards the patient. According to some nurses whom I have taught, one of the difficulties in trying to understand the language of ethics, for example, moral obligations such as 'respect for autonomy' and 'beneficence' is their evaluative nature. Perhaps then this difficulty, in comprehending the evaluative nature of moral language, is one reason why they rely instead on personal qualities, intuition and instinct in moral decision-making.

Moral sensitivity

To be sensitive to a person's needs suggests that one is able to identify the other's needs perhaps more easily than another person is able to. The phrase 'morally sensitive' connotes a positive and admirable quality, one that in nurses suggests that care will be morally good. In contrast, if I am insensitive to my patient's feelings then I might fail to perceive his feelings and as a result, I might act as though his feelings do not matter to me. To be a morally sensitive nurse, it is insufficient to merely perceive patients' needs. One's perceptions ought to produce a morally appropriate response; perceptions also help to form one's moral motives. According to the virtue-based approach to morality, one should respond to another person's interests and needs in morally good ways. Nurses should act, think and feel from the virtues including honesty, kindness, trustworthiness, respectfulness and courage. Take kindness as an example. Acting kindly towards a patient is an example of acting well. But as noted earlier, the virtues motivate thoughts and feelings too and these clearly affect how one responds to someone else. Kind thoughts and feelings are morally good, and kind responses towards patients tend to have positive effects on their ability to survive illness and then recover and fare well. Sensitivity towards patients' interests and needs and reflection on the morally relevant features can be seen as moral sensitivity. The opposite – lack of moral sensitivity or moral insensitivity – can manifest itself in various ways including, for example, the lack of insight that some nurses demonstrate towards patients for instance in relation to allowing a patient some privacy and nurses apparently oblivious to the need for patients to have time alone with their loved ones. In my view, it is a false assumption to believe that all nurses are morally sensitive to patients' interests and needs in particular their distress. One of the major aims of current nurse education is to develop morally sensitive practitioners.[19] Being morally sensitive might include the notion of being empathetic[20] or having fellow feeling for another person's needs. It seems to me that one component of displaying moral sensitivity is one's ability to assimilate information – clinical and moral – and interpret it to provide help for a patient and respond in morally good ways, i.e., acting from the virtues. The context and particulars of each situation need to be taken into account and given considerable thought. The ability of nurses to think about a wide range of notions, including patients' characters, interests and needs is important to being sensitive. However, it is not sufficient for nurses to merely ask questions in an attempt to gather important information (even this endeavour is more difficult than it might first appear).[21] To develop moral sensitivity, it is crucial that nurses make sense of this information.

Several authors have drawn attention to the important role played by emotion in the moral life generally and in moral thinking in particular. Oakley[22] states that emotions are felt experiences composed of desires and cognitions that are manifested towards others. Emotions, for example, sympathy, compassion and empathy are sometimes held to be synonymous with the virtues. However, on the conception of a virtue that I presented in Chapter 3, compassion is a virtue but sympathy and empathy[23] are not virtues. One of the central aims of the virtue-based approach to morality is to promote nurses' morally virtuous acts, thoughts and feelings; or to put it another way, nurses ought to respond to patients' emotions in morally virtuous ways (this is one reason why I examined some common emotions experienced by ill patients in Chapter 2).

Moral imagination

Scott[24] has examined the idea of 'imaginative identification'. In her words:

> For example, I may become angry with my mother due to certain comments she makes and directs, unfairly in my view, at my husband (who is present during the scenario). However I suggest that the anger is a direct response to my perception of the hurt/embarrassment I might feel if I were my husband listening to the comments.[25]

Empathy seems to be related to the activity of imagination or at least imagination involves being empathetic; perhaps empathy is a necessary but not sufficient component of imagination. It seems to me that the activity of moral imagination requires one to put oneself in another person's position (as Scott did above). Questions include 'How would I feel if that cruel comment was said about me?' and 'How would I feel if the nurse spoke to me in such a callous way?' In relation to moral imagination and the moral life, Murdoch[26] believes that one sees that which confronts one by attending properly, by looking selflessly and completely. The objects of such attention include things of value such as virtuous people and the notion of goodness itself. Nurses ought to think hard about the virtues and vices and imagine how traits such as compassion and patience will motivate morally good interpersonal responses.

The virtue-based helping relationship

When nurses cultivate and act from the virtues, I shall call the resulting relationship a virtue-based helping relationship. Nurses will need to exercise a broad range of different moral virtues in order to respond to patients' interests and needs in morally good ways. Examples of moral virtues important in the development and sustenance of a morally good helping relationship are compassion (including benevolence or kind-ness), courage, respectfulness, patience, tolerance, justice, trustworthi-ness and honesty. Regarding the first three virtues, I suggest that the virtue of compassion is the moral foundation of the helping relation-ship between nurse and patient, courage is a moral virtue needed to be an effective patient advocate and respectfulness is one of the virtues necessary to empower patients. The list above is clearly not exhaustive; different virtues will be implicated depending on the role and aims of the nurse, the patient's interests and needs and the range of morally rel-evant features considered important in each situation. The fact that the pivotal focus might be on one virtue, for example, compassion, does not mean that others such as justice will be neglected.

The virtue of compassion

In this section, I aim to examine the virtue of compassion. What does compassion consist of? What exactly is a nurse saying when she describes a colleague as compassionate? These questions can be applied to all moral virtues and if responses to the questions are inadequate, then critics will object to the virtue-based approach to morality on the grounds that it is insufficient. It seems to me unsatis-factory to say 'John, a staff nurse, needs to show compassion to his patients' if (a) John does not know what it means to show compassion and (b) John's colleague, Sandra, understands compassion in a different way to John; hence they each respond to patients in perhaps different ways. Compassion is a common notion in nursing (I use 'notion' because compassion is often referred to as a dimension or faculty needed by nurses). Kinion et al. simply state that nurses 'must show compassion';[27] however, this command suggests an underlying deontic reason for showing compassion. Furthermore, instead of presenting a conception of compassion Kinion et al. merely cite the term once at the end of the article.

In what ways should one with compassion act? According to Blum compassion 'requires the disposition to perform beneficent actions'.[28] Thus, the actions of a compassionate nurse will benefit the patient and as noted in Chapter 7, actions can benefit people in both physical and non-physical ways. The nurses in a recent Delphi[29] questionnaire study believed that kindness (or benevolence[30]) is a component of compas-sion, thus kind acts, thoughts and feelings are part of being a compas-sionate nurse. What about motives? A compassionate nurse's motive for action is internal, i.e., the virtue of compassion forms part of one's identity and it is a character trait that shows other people the kind of nurse one is. Because of these internal dispositions and motives, being compassionate is a natural response for the compassionate nurse. Besides a moral dimension, Pellegrino and Thomasma claim that compassion includes an intellectual dimension

> it consists in the disposition habitually to comprehend, assess, and weigh the uniqueness of this patient's predicament of illness.[31]

This point relates directly to the discussion in Chapter 2 concerning patients' lived experience of illness and nurses being motivated to listen to patients' narrative accounts of illness.

The virtues in particular compassion, but also benevolence and honesty developed as an important pattern of interest throughout the Delphi study[32] noted above. This three-round questionnaire study aimed to examine how mental health nurses make moral decisions. Compassion was given 16 diverse meanings; this finding is unsurprising given its phenomenological complexity. Ambiguity and uncertainty are to be expected in qualitative research findings because nurses are individuals with particular views about morality and nursing practice. In this Delphi study, compassion was understood to include components of benevolence, kindness, caring and empathy. Some of the 16 meanings of compassion were 'show understanding about how they [the patients] are feeling/behaving', 'compassion is caring and showing it' and 'give time and listen'. A subsequent question asked is: 'Is behaving and acting compassionately important to the goal of being an ethical psychiatric nurse?' More than 70% of the sample responded in the affirmative to this question. Responses included:

> I think behaving and acting compassionately is a goal of being a human but particularly for nurses, caring for vulnerable people.

Some nurses were uncertain about this question, for example,

> for the most part, behaving and acting compassionately is a major part of a psychiatric nurse's role, but in some instances this may not be appropriate.

Another nurse answered in the negative to this question, saying:

> On occasions, because of my professional attitudes and position, despite not always feeling compassionate, I can fulfil this goal.

In Chapter 2, I examined the feeling of vulnerability that patients often experience. For the nurse in the first quote, being compassionate is necessary because of such vulnerability. Two points need noting regarding the second and third quotes above. In relation to the second quote, there is the question of the appropriateness of one's feelings and emotions. This is a difficult issue that in part concerns whether nurses believe they should be 'patient-focused' or 'task-focused'. Nurses might worry that being patient-focused necessarily means forming close relationships with patients, and such nurses might fear that forming excessively close relationships go beyond the boundaries of a 'professional' nurse–patient relationship and might jeopardize the 'ethical' status of the nurse. In this Delphi study, several nurses mentioned this point, describing colleagues as 'unethical' if they formed 'overly close' relationships. My second point is in relation to the third quote above. It is not clear what this nurse means by 'professional attitudes and position'. On a positive note, this nurse is honest in admitting that sometimes she lacks compassion for a particular patient. Despite this, she believes that she can still be an 'ethical' nurse. This response helps to bring out an important distinction between actions and feelings. On the one hand, this nurse acting probably from the obligation of beneficence benefits the patient, for example, she administers a psychotropic medication that reduces the patient's mania. This action is clearly beneficent. But on the other hand, this action is according to the nurse carried out without the *feeling* of compassion or without the nurse *being* compassionate. The nurse's motive is one of obligation instead of virtue. It is plain to see that actions can be beneficent but in terms of motive, character traits and the quality of the interpersonal response this is very different from acting, thinking and feeling from the virtues. According to Lutzen and Barbosa da Silva,[33] compassion is an active virtue; others include courage and trust. Active virtues 'motivate the agent to the appropriate action in order to help the dependent patient'.[34] Being a compassionate nurse will involve such things as wishing to understand what is troubling a patient, wanting to spend time with a patient, listening to a patient's lived experience of the illness and asking the patient questions so that the nurse can make some sense of the patient's lived experience. Showing compassion helps to develop a bond between patients and nurses and if the latter act, think and feel in compassionate ways then the helping relationship will be promoted. Moreover, exercising compassion tends to promote other virtues such as trustworthiness and justice.[35] This description of compassion has established a picture of what a compassionate nurse is like, what she feels and does. However, I realize that it is not easy to identify, cultivate and habitually exercise the virtues, let alone do so for morally good reasons. Compassion is no exception as Nouwen et al. suggest:

> Compassion asks us to go where it hurts, to enter into places of pain, to share in brokenness, fear, confusion and anguish ... compassion means full immersion in the condition of being human.[36]

In Chapter 3, I conceived a moral virtue as an admirable character trait, deserving praise and admiration from others that is habitually exercised and helps its possessor and others to fare well in life. Based on this conception, I view compassion as a moral virtue.[37] Compassion is an example of an other-regarding or altruistic[38] virtue because typically the exercise of compassion helps others to a greater degree than its possessor. Compassion is a moral virtue needed by nurses to develop and sustain a helping relationship between themselves and patients, and compassionate care is an example of morally excellent and 'successful'[39] care.

Compassion and caring

What is the relationship between caring and compassion? The terms 'caring' and 'care' have been used several times in this book, and the notion of 'caring' appears to be fundamentally important in nursing and it is necessary to describe the work of nurses. However, the concept of caring is poorly conceptualized; it is difficult to move past a basic understanding, for example, 'it's what nurses do'. A distinction has been made between 'caring for' and 'caring about'.[40] The former suggests a deontic motive, a more distanced type of caring where the care is per- haps not 'patient–focused'. 'Caring about' sounds more inclusive, a more developed and wide-ranging form of care where the carer focuses on a diverse set of concerns. And as noted in Chapter 3, Barker talks about 'caring with', which suggests a collaborative sense of caring. I believe that 'caring' represents an attitude about someone or some- thing in the world. For example, 'I care for Carol' or 'I care about music'. The meaning attributed to the term 'care' is usually a positive one. For instance, if I overheard someone on a bus saying 'John cares a lot for Sally' without knowing anything about John, I might assume that John was a good, caring person. In other words, the term 'care' produces a positive response in others. But I suggest that because care is an attitu- dinal term, it needs qualifying to bring out its real meaning; remember that according to one of the nurses who participated in the afore- mentioned Delphi study,[41] it is possible to care *without* compassion.

On reflection, I can recall nurses who went about their work efficiently but I do not remember seeing compassionate care from these nurses. I suggest that the terms 'care' and 'caring' need to be supplemented by other terms; indeed I think that in many cases the addition of a virtue term will clarify the meaning. For example, 'I care *justly* about Sam' or 'I am caring *patiently* for Jake'; perhaps if a virtue term does not make sense then an adjective or adverb might, for instance, 'John cares *passionately* for Sally'. It should be clear that I reject the claim that caring is a virtue.[42] I believe that caring is not a morally admirable character trait that helps its possessor and others to fare well. Rather it represents an attitude about someone or something in the world. Furthermore, I reject the idea that 'care' is sufficient for leading morally good lives because simply put, it is possible to care in ways that are not morally good.

I shall now briefly describe the important role played by another two moral virtues, namely, courage and respectfulness.

Courage and advocacy

There is a rich body of literature on the notion of advocacy and the role of the nurse as patient advocate.[43] According to obligation-based moral theories, nurses ought to act from the obligations of beneficence and respect for patients' autonomy, and an important aspect of these obligations is the requirement for nurses to promote and protect patients' interests and needs. Being an advocate for a patient can involve putting the interests of the patient ahead of one's own, for example, defending and promoting the wishes of a patient with cancer when these oppose the views put forward by the consultant.[44] Nurses who act as advocates can depending upon the precise circumstances leave themselves vulnerable to professional dispute and emotional distress. Therefore one of the virtues needed to be a successful advocate is courage; perhaps we should refer to it as 'moral courage'. People need courage to get through life because courage helps one to endure the hostilities that daily life can provide. In general, people need to exercise courage for self-protection.[45] But possessing courage does not come naturally to many people. Cultivating and exercising courage means that nurses really *want* to help patients in distress. Without such altruistic desires, nurses would be far less inclined to put themselves in the potentially vulnerable and dangerous position that being an advocate can demand. I shall not discuss the moral arguments for and against nurses acting as advocates for patients. Suffice it to say that there are good reasons why nurses are not suitably placed to make effective advocates.[46] Despite these arguments, it remains clear that a nurse will at least on some occasions wish to act as an advocate for a patient. If this is so, then the nurse will require the virtue of courage in order to be an effective advocate and help to protect and promote the patient's interests and needs. But we have seen that traditional accounts of consequentialism and deontology fail to discuss the important role played by moral virtues and as such, the role of courage will be neglected. This is a major oversight because acting from obligation is not sufficient for morally excellent nursing practice in general and being a morally good (successful) patient advocate in particular.

Respectfulness and empowerment

As noted in Chapter 2, the notion of empowerment is heavily debated in the literature. However, the debate tends not to describe (let alone examine) the sorts of character traits required by nurses for empowering patients. I suggest that nurses will not be able to empower patients if they lack traits of character such as respectfulness (I also suggest that nurses require other important virtues to empower patients, for example, patience and tolerance). From an obligation-based moral perspective, patients will be empowered if nurses act from the obligations of respect for autonomy and beneficence. However, while these obligations might provide a degree of action guidance especially for novice nurses, it remains crucial to examine the moral virtues and their role in empowering patients. The fundamental point is that nurses are not robots and the manner in which obligations are perceived, interpreted and applied concerns the kind of person one is. Nurses can examine the virtue of respectfulness and they can appreciate the kinds of actions, thoughts and feelings fostered by this virtue. For example, a nurse approaches a patient with asthma because she sees that his hands are shaking more than usual. The nurse listens attentively to the patient's narrative and relays this information to the doctor. As a result, the patient is prescribed a reduced dosage of vasodilator, which was causing the shakes. The patient feels physically better, but he also feels more empowered.

In the next section, I conceive 'the virtue-based approach to moral decision-making' in nursing practice. This approach consists of three features: first, the exercise of moral virtues; second, the use of judgement; and third, the use of moral wisdom. Virtue ethics addresses the first feature, i.e., acting from the virtues. Henceforth, when I refer to the virtue-based approach, I am referring to a strong action-guiding version of virtue ethics in tandem with the use of judgement and moral wisdom.

The virtue-based approach to moral decision-making in nursing practice

The virtue of compassion

Imagine a nurse who is caring for a male patient with Parkinson's disease (PD). Because this disease affects neuromuscular transmission, problems of living result, for example, the patient will need help with activities of living such as washing, dressing, eating and walking. Jack has PD and lives alone at home; he has a daily visit by a community nurse. Jack's favourite nurse is Carol because he believes that Carol understands him better than the other nurses and he thinks that unlike some other nurses, Carol is a kind nurse who shows him compassion. Carol is disposed to carry out beneficent actions that help Jack; she tries hard to meet Jack's needs including his emotional needs. Although Carol has a busy daily schedule, she enjoys spending time with Jack and takes an interest in his life; for example, she asks him if the new Sinemet medication is working and if the carers have done his shopping. Conversing with Jack is often time consuming because his speech is usually slurred. Another reason why Jack likes Carol is that he regards Carol as a very patient nurse and in this respect she is different from many other nurses who rush him. Carol wants to get to know Jack well so that she can understand his illness and its effects on his life, and as a result she hopes to help Jack live with PD, for example, by managing his muscle tremors[47] more effectively. Carol is motivated from deep inside to show kindness to her patients; her parents and friends describe her as a genuinely kind person. Kindness is, for Carol, one of the core values of being a good nurse. Carol aims to better understand Jack's predicament; she thinks about him before she visits and when she leaves Jack's house, she imagines what it would be like to be unable to walk more than 10 metres without tumbling to the floor, what it might be like dribbling when trying to eat and what it might be like to be unable to get dressed nearly every morning of one's life. Carol is motivated to be compassionate *not* because other people tell her to be so or because the NMC code of conduct[48] demands her to be. Instead Carol is habitually kind because it is part of who she is as a person. Carol believes that patients such as Jack fare better when she is kind. This scenario is not meant to read as a caricature of a caring patient-focused nurse although I realize it is a caricature. It seems to me that one of the central points regarding so-called holistic and patient-centred nursing care is that for these notions to mean something nurses ought to exercise the moral virtues. An aim of the 'Carol and Jack' scenario is to show

how it is possible for a nurse to think about the meaning of compassion and apply it to the care of her patients. Moreover, besides the consequences and nature of actions the virtue-based approach takes into account the importance of one's emotions and feelings in the moral life. Carol demonstrates compassion towards Jack and she is also patient towards him; she understands the effects that PD can have on Jack, for example, the fact that it often takes him a long time before he is able to speak. It is important to clarify that a nurse who acts from the virtues is highly unlikely to act from a single virtue; this scenario helps to show how altruistic virtues such as compassion and patience are interrelated.

The use of judgement and moral wisdom in nursing practice

The virtue-based approach to moral decision-making in nursing practice acknowledges and encourages the use of judgement and moral wisdom, i.e., moral perception, moral sensitivity and moral imagination. Suppose Carol visits Jack one morning as usual. However, this morning Jack does not wish to get out of bed; Carol observes him for signs of pain and discomfort. She asks him whether he slept well, but Jack replies that muscle tremors and spasms stopped him from sleeping. Jack asks Carol if he can remain in bed for an hour or two longer; however, Carol is concerned that Jack may develop a sacral pressure sore as his skin is already very red. Having perceived Jack's distress, Carol thinks carefully about how she should respond to Jack's needs. On the one hand, he wants to sleep for another hour or two and this is important given his lack of sleep. But on the other hand, Carol does not wish Jack to develop a pressure sore that will cause him further physical and emotional distress. Carol thinks about how she would feel in similar circumstances and she thinks about the wide range of morally relevant features that I described earlier (see p. 127). Carol thinks about this information, the knowledge she has of Jack's condition and her understanding of Jack as a person; through this process, Carol is able to make a judgement. Carol decides to ask Jack if she can move his position in the bed and she explains to Jack the risk of pressure sore development. Jack understands this risk; they mutually agree that Jack will lie on his left side for a couple of hours. Carol contacts a carer and asks her to visit Jack in approximately two hours. Before Carol leaves she gives Jack an additional dose of Sinemet[49] to relieve his distressing muscle tremors. Later in the day, the carer tells Carol that Jack was much happier because his spasms abated and he managed to sleep for an hour or so. It has been noted how the virtue-based approach to morality does not overfocus on actions. Instead it acknowledges and examines the importance of the thoughts and feelings of patients and nurses in the moral life; in short, it aims to help patients fare well. In order to discover a wide range of ways to help patients through and beyond illness, the virtue-based approach encourages the use of reflection. Being virtuous, for example, kind, promotes the ability of the nurse to reflect on a wide range of nursing and medical interventions. While the obligation-based approach to morality does not necessarily preclude this kind of reasoning, the virtue-based approach places the emphasis on a wider range of morally important features, promotes the development of a helping nurse–patient relationship and fosters reflection on the interests and needs of patients. If nurses' moral motives are limited to obligations, then the moral virtues and the nurses' and patients' thoughts and feelings are more likely to be ignored. If a nurse focuses on *only* the consequences or nature of acts/omissions, then it seems to me that she is limiting the range of practices and activities that in some way might help a patient. An example might help. Suppose a patient has chronic back pain that is secondary to cancer. The virtue-based approach to morality encourages the nurse to use moral wisdom – moral perception, sensitivity and imagination – to reveal information about the patient that might otherwise remain unknown. In this case, the nurse spends considerable time[50] with the patient evaluating his pain and the effectiveness of the prescribed morphine. By acting from the virtue-based approach, it becomes clear that the patient's pain is not well controlled plus the nurse discovers that the patient is suffering from severe constipation.[51] The nurse is intent on helping the patient to fare well through the cancer both the disease itself and its treatment. She therefore conveys to the doctor that the patient's pain is poorly controlled and that he is suffering from constipation. The nurse makes it clear to the medic how much distress the patient is in. The morphine is soon replaced with Fentanyl[52] that proves more effective in controlling the patient's pain and re-establishing regular bowel movements. It is sometimes not possible – perhaps because of the high intensity of the work and an insufficient number of nurses – to spend a lot of time getting to know a patient. Spending time with patients might be possible, but we have already seen that literature shows that nurses spend minimal time in direct contact with patients. Hence, it is morally admirable for the nurse in this example to act, think and feel from the virtues of patience and kindness. The impact of the virtues is clear to see: this nurse was able to promote the patient's quality of life and I suggest that this kind of intervention is the kind of intervention that many patients remember.

Merits of the virtue-based approach to moral decision-making in nursing practice

In Chapters 3 and 5, I examined some of the merits of the virtues and virtue ethics from the perspective of general ethics. In this chapter, I have considered other merits of this approach, for example, how it promotes the use of judgement and moral wisdom, and how these morally important features can help nurses make morally good judgements. I shall now summarize and if necessary clarify these important merits.

First, nurses utilize the language of the virtues and vices on a daily basis. For example, words such as 'care', 'fair', 'well', 'just' and 'good' are all aretaic terms.[53] It therefore seems sensible to claim that the language used by nurses in practice should be utilized in the moral theory that they adopt to guide their practice. Second, the aforementioned point is more important than it might at first appear. Supported in part by Hursthouse's[54] v-rules thesis (see Chapter 5) aretaic terms like the above actually do provide a good degree of action-guidance. In other words by thinking hard about words such as 'kind', nurses can get a sense of which actions kind nurses ought to perform. For instance, Tom is 15 years old and bored having been in traction on an orthopaedic ward for six weeks. I begin to think about the meaning of 'kindness' and I bring to mind several examples of kind deeds. From conversing with Tom, I know that he enjoys reading music magazines and within a couple of hours, I have managed to find a few relevant magazines from the hospital library. When I visit Tom with the magazines, he appears genuinely surprised and grateful and he thanks me for my kindness and thoughtfulness. Therefore through reflection, the sorts of actions, thoughts and feelings that aretaic words can conjure up in one's imagination become quite clear. It was noted in Chapter 5 that virtue ethics is charged with being unable to provide adequate action-guidance and this criticism is held to be a serious flaw of virtue ethics and the pivotal reason why a strong version of virtue ethics is held to be non-viable (see Chapter 5). To reiterate, I reject this claim and I assert that a strong virtue ethics – one that provides adequate action-guidance for nurses – is both possible and plausible. As such, it ought to be acknowledged that it provides a serious moral alternative to the traditional obligation-based moral theories of consequentialism and deontology. Third, despite criticisms to the contrary the virtue-based approach to morality does not minimize the crucial notion of consequences in the moral life of patients and nurses; as noted in Chapter 4, the idea of an action's consequences/outcomes is fundamentally important in everyday life. The virtue-based approach recognizes this fact. However, the virtue-based approach does not over-focus on the importance of an action's consequences at the expense of other morally important features; indeed the virtue-based approach examines several features of morality ignored by obligation-based moral theories. Several of these features were discussed in Chapter 5. Fourth, an example of a morally relevant feature taken into account by the virtue-based approach is the important role played by emotions such as distress, fear, anxiety, vulnerability, guilt and remorse in the moral life of nurses and patients. One of the main points here is that it is morally appropriate for nurses to *feel* these kinds of emotions in their daily work. Such emotions are often distressing and unpleasant, for example, a nurse withholds information from a patient with terminal illness because the patient's relatives believe she could not cope and second, a nurse lies to a paralyzed patient when asked if he will ever walk again because the nurse cannot bear to tell the patient to whom she is close that he will never walk again. In both examples it is morally appropriate for the nurse involved to feel certain emotions including, for example, guilt, anxiety and regret; perhaps some of these emotions are felt because the nurse involved is worried about how the patient will respond upon hearing the truth. Because the emphasis of the virtue-based approach is not solely on actions, it takes emotions and feelings into account and recognizes their contribution to the moral lives of patients and nurses. Fifth, partly because of the distinction noted by Hursthouse[55] in Chapter 4 between two possible ways of using the phrases 'right moral decision/morally right action' the virtue-based approach does not assume that all moral dilemmas are resolvable; so it does not seek to resolve moral dilemmas. Instead of the major aim being to reveal the 'right thing to do', one of the central aims of the virtue-based approach is to promote acting well, i.e., acting from the virtues. Regarding nurses involved in moral dilemmas, for example, when a patient is coerced into having ECT against his wishes, the morally appropriate response from a virtuous nurse is to feel moral remainder principally because involvement in such distressing situations should produce certain emotional responses in a nurse. In the example of ECT, the nurse might feel regret and remorse for some of the things she said and did. Furthermore as noted in Chapter 4, in even more terrible situations which Hursthouse calls 'irresolvable' and 'tragic' dilemmas the lives of those involved including nurses and patients will often end up being marred in some way. Traditional accounts of consequentialism and deontology neglect this morally important feature and are therefore incomplete and inadequate moral theories. For a nursing ethics to be complete and plausible, it needs to take the role of emotions and moral remainder into account, and in my view this is one of the most notable reasons why the virtue-based approach to morality is a more convincing nursing ethics than its deontic competitors. Sixth, the question of how to educate the young to be good persons is clearly an important one. In nursing, it is necessary to consider how student nurses can develop to be morally good nurses. Rather strangely, the obligation-based approach fails to sufficiently debate these questions; instead it is almost as though people of all ages just *will* act in accordance with moral obligations. In contrast, the virtue-based approach asks questions concerning the moral education of the young and in examining such issues as learning from role models and the habituation of moral (and clinical) excellences, it provides a good starting point for further exploration of issues concerning the moral education of nurses (I discuss the topic of moral education further in the 'Conclusions'). Seventh, the virtue-based approach to morality promotes a narrative account of a patient's lived experience of illness. As previously noted, patients feel a range of emotions including fear, anxiety, powerlessness and vulnerability and the virtue-based approach recognizes the presence of such emotions. Illness creates these emotions and these can be intensified through the process of hospitalization. It seems to me that the virtue-based approach recognizes and promotes the ideal of patient-centred and holistic care. Literature was examined in Chapter 2 that indicates that (at least) some patients and some patients' relatives define 'high-' quality care in terms that I would call virtue-based care. For example, high- or good-quality care involves nurses being gentle, patient, honest and kind towards patients. I believe that good nursing care and the exercise of the moral virtues is synonymous. Eighth, in my view one of the most notable merits of the virtue-based approach to morality is its acceptance and promotion of the use of judgement and moral wisdom in moral decision-making. Earlier in this chapter, I examined both judgement and the associated notion of moral wisdom and applied it to nursing practice. While deontological moral rules are useful, conflicts frequently occur. Nurses should perceive and assimilate precise pieces of information and examine some of the specifics within morally complex situations; judgement is required to work through this assemblage of information. Moral wisdom – moral perception, moral sensitivity and moral imagination – is utilized in tandem with judgement in an attempt to make morally good decisions. While this is problematic (I will discuss criticisms later in this chapter), the virtue-based approach, unlike obligation-based moral theories, construes moral decision-making as difficult. In this respect, the virtue-based approach describes and reflects more accurately the work of clinical nurses including the innumerable morally complex dilemmas and conflicts between obligations that arise daily in contemporary nursing practice.

The virtue-based approach and reasons for action

Another merit of the virtue-based approach namely 'reasons for action' requires specific discussion. 'Reasons for action' is a richly documented philosophical topic[56] and from a virtue-based perspective, Hursthouse has examined this topic and the associated topic of moral motivation in relation to abortion.[57] Usually, the morality of abortion is discussed by adopting a framework of moral rights. However as Hursthouse claims 'in exercising a moral right, I can do something cruel, or callous, or selfish, … inconsiderate, … dishonest'.[58] In other words, people can exercise their rights viciously. Pregnancy and childbirth are very important states of being for many (though not all) women. According to Hursthouse it is important to recognize and contextualize pregnancy and childbirth within the whole narrative of a woman's life. The woman's interests, needs, values and life plans need to be identified and taken into account in decision-making. Aborting a foetus might be a morally kind act for a woman who never wanted children if after prolonged deliberation she feels strongly that she could not give a child a caring and happy environment in which to live well. Acting from kindness is an example of acting morally well. Conversely, a woman's reason for wanting an abortion might turn on selfishness, for example, a woman states: 'I want an abortion because I want to continue shopping and having a child would spoil my enjoyment of life.' Or perhaps the reason for action might be dishonesty, for instance, 'I want an abortion because the father of the child is not my husband and I don't want my husband to find out'. This kind of reasoning can be applied to nursing practice, for example, a patient refusing her medications. It seems to me that one of the many strengths of the virtue-based approach is that it promotes an examination of the particulars of each situation. In this example the patient might refuse to take her antidepressants because they make her feel very tired. The patient is really keen to write a letter to a friend thanking her for a recent present. It is several days since the present arrived but the patient's depression prevented her from writing a letter. She is now in a rush to write and post the letter, but the antidepressants make her feel very tired and have affected her ability to concentrate on specific tasks. This is the reason why the patient does not want to take her medications. Her motive is that she wants to demonstrate gratitude to one of her closest friends, someone she has known for 30 years. The patient values loyalty and she wishes to remain friends with this person. Essentially, the patient's reasons for refusing the medications are grounded in the virtues of gratitude, respectfulness and loyalty.

Criticisms of the virtue-based approach to moral decision-making in nursing practice

In Chapters 3 and 5, I noted some important criticisms of the virtues and virtue ethics. I shall now explore these criticisms in the context of contemporary nursing practice. First, it was noted in Chapter 3 that an assumption is made regarding moral virtues being morally good traits of character, for example, that it is morally good to be honest. The claim that a specific character trait is a virtue will be put forward because it meets a certain conception of a virtue; the authorities for such conceptions include several of Western philosophy's most respected thinkers, for example, Aristotle,[59] Slote[60] and Hursthouse.[61] I am not saying that each conception is *necessarily* well argued; one needs to consider whether the character trait under investigation satisfies the criteria outlined in the conception. My conception was given in Chapter 3: a virtue is a character trait that is habitually performed, which disposes the possessor to act, think and feel in morally good ways, and the possessor deserves praise and admiration from others. Moral virtues are valuable for several reasons not least because exercising moral virtues will typically have a positive impact on the lives of patients. Furthermore in Chapter 2, it was noted that empirical research indicates that patients *feel* virtuous care, for instance, the kindness of a nurse. Moreover, it was also noted that some patient's perceptions of 'high-' and 'good-' quality care equate with nurses exercising moral virtues. Second, it is possible that some people might believe that the language of the virtues is old fashioned. For example, if one is described as 'virtuous' then it might be understood to mean 'prissy' or 'prudish'. This interpretation might deter people in particular nurses from learning more about the virtues and the virtue-based approach to morality. Clearly, there is a great need to teach the virtue-based approach in nurse education and unfortunately, evidence suggests that sometimes this does not happen.[62] Part of the reason why the virtues might be seen as prudish and old fashioned is because of the history of nursing especially the influence of Nightingale who wanted nurses to be good, with high moral character. The pivotal virtues in Nightingale's era included obedience and subservience because the nurse's role consisted in following doctors' orders. In contemporary nursing ethics, the pivotal virtues are caring virtues such as compassion and benevolence; this dramatic difference in emphasis helps to demonstrate how candidates for the status of virtues change over time. It is possible that some people still think of the virtues – if indeed, they think about them at all – as submissive traits of character; if this is true, then it seems to me that this is more reason to educate nurses about the virtues.

Third, the charge of moral relativism can be levelled at the virtue-based approach to morality. It is alleged that since virtues are human character traits it follows that disagreement will arise in identifying which traits are virtues. I accept that people will produce lists of different virtues, which will happen, in part, because human interests, needs and values are distinct. Because of the complexity of human lives, I find it difficult to accept that an advocate of the virtue-based approach would lead his life according to *just* one virtue. Irrespective of whether a specific virtue such as justice is considered fundamentally important to the moral life, it seems to me that the importance of other moral virtues will be realized. This is a feature of the virtue-based approach; because human lives are complex and multifaceted many different virtues will be necessary to lead morally good lives. I accept that people might prioritize virtues differently, for instance, one person might think that kindness is more important than patience. People prioritize the importance of moral obligations differently; it was noted in Chapter 4 that 'respect for autonomy' appears now to be the predominant moral obligation especially in the current climate of empowering patients. Likewise some people might believe in a 'fundamental' virtue such as justice. The point is that certain virtues will be more appropriate and applicable than others depending on several factors, including one's role and the particulars of each situation. Imagine that there are ten nurses on a medical ward. Some people might assume that all ten nurses would agree that compassion and honesty are key virtues that ought to be exercised in the nurse–patient relationship. But I believe that this assumption would be overly optimistic. Why should ten different people with their own unique values about nursing practice agree on something so complicated? Instead, I would expect some disagreement; for example, five nurses agree that compassion and honesty are really important virtues, three nurses claim that respectfulness is a crucial virtue while the remaining two nurses disagree among themselves and fail to reach any firm conclusions. Through debate, it is agreed that all of these virtues should be demonstrated in the delivery of patient care. Consensus is also reached on the view that some virtues will be more important than others depending on several issues such as the nature of the nursing activity, the patient's interests and needs and the kind of nurse one wishes to be in a given interaction. I reject the claim that disagreement would cause insurmountable problems. In the same way that there is disagreement concerning the moral importance of the four principles, it seems to me that identifying and prioritizing different virtues is not necessarily problematic for nurses.

Why should nurses be virtuous when nursing patients who have committed deplorable acts?

This question is particularly important. It raises serious issues regarding why nurses ought to act from the virtues. I shall therefore explore this question in some detail. Examples of deplorable acts include rape and child abuse. Rapists and child abusers often come into contact with forensic psychiatrists and nurses. The deontic approach, for example, the four principles approach, instructs nurses to abide by certain moral obligations. Such moral demands ought to apply irrespective of what acts patients have carried out. For example, the obligation of beneficence means that nurses are obliged to benefit and do good for patients. This obligation should be fulfilled whether nurses like and admire the patient or whether nurses dislike and are repulsed by the patient. On the face of it, this idea appears to be reasonable. However, in terms of one's feelings it is far from simple to *always* meet such strict moral demands. As previously noted, one of the difficulties with the obligation-based approach to morality is that moral obligations provide moral agents with an external motive for action. However, if the nurse does not *feel* benevolent towards the patient because she is angry with and repulsed by the patient then it is not going to be easy for her to act from beneficence. We compare and evaluate each other's acts, thoughts and feelings and it seems to me that this is a natural part of being human. If we judge someone's actions to be deplorable, then it fails to make sense to like and admire the perpetrator of such actions. Rape and child abuse are examples of horrendous, vicious crimes that violate human rights. I suggest that the vast majority of people believe that rape and child abuse are deplorable acts and as such, the perpetrators of these crimes might be despised for their actions.

I shall make four claims in response to the question: 'Why should nurses be virtuous when nursing patients who have committed deplorable acts?' First, when people describe acts such as rape and child abuse as *deplorable* and the perpetrator as *despicable* it is the aretaic language of the virtues, and in these examples the vices, which people utilize. These terms describe someone's moral character. Instead of admiring or praising someone for displaying the virtues, it is natural to believe that rapists and child abusers ought to be despised (of course, it is possible to argue that while these *actions* ought to be despised this is not the same as despising the actors). Such aretaic terms are as Hursthouse[63] and Benn[64] claim common in everyday language and these terms are useful because they provide a rich degree of descriptive power; this is not the case with the language of the deontic approach. It is possible to argue that the use of such aretaic terms is (for at least some people) cathartic, i.e., it can facilitate the relief of raw and potentially negative emotions such as anger and hatred in nurses who are obliged to care for rapists and child abusers. My second response is related to the first. It is that the virtue-based approach to morality recognizes the importance of the emotions in the moral life of both patients and nurses. In contrast, traditional accounts of consequentialism and deontology fail to sufficiently take the emotions of nurses into account. As noted above, nurses might feel a range of strong emotions such as anger, hatred, rage and perhaps even vengeance. Such emotions are brushed aside or simply considered 'unethical' or 'wrong'. My third response is brief; it is that in nursing people who have carried out despicable and evil deeds we are reminded of the dark side of humanity. We are presented with an extremely vivid picture of the vicious side of human nature in particular the terrible deeds that people are capable of doing. Although this is not a positive realization, this fact about human nature provides further reason to investigate the merits of the virtue-based approach to morality. My final response regarding this serious question is not intended to defend the despicable and deplorable acts committed by perpetrators of rape and child abuse. However, it is a response that I believe the virtue-based approach would make because it centres on reasons for action. The essential point is that despite the inherent difficulty, nurses should try to understand why some people perform deplorable deeds, i.e., ideally we should aim to identify and examine the perpetrator's motives and reasons for action. For example, perhaps the abuser was abused as a child or perhaps there is evidence of mental illness and/or diminished responsibility. The virtue-based approach claims that people ought to cultivate the virtues although this requires hard work and determination. Might it then be possible for some of these perpetrators to change their characters if they received morally virtuous and clinically effective treatment? I remain, however, uncertain about the empirical evidence that might support or deny this possibility. Perhaps some forensic nurses would reply with: 'Only someone who has never cared for perpetrators of rape and child abuse would say something like that.' Nevertheless, it is a view that, I think, the virtue-based approach to morality would advocate, and I think that specific virtues would include compassion and kindness. Supporters of the slippery slope argument might ask: 'Where are the boundaries to be drawn if nurses (and other health care practitioners) were allowed to treat patients as they liked?' For example, is it morally justifiable for a homophobic nurse to refuse to care for a homosexual man? Or is it morally justifiable for a racist Caucasian to refuse to care for an African-American? If we were allowed to practice according to our unchecked moral values, what does that say about the virtue and obligation of justice?

The problem of exercising a virtue to an excessive degree

Aristotle's 'doctrine of the mean' is sometimes taken to mean that people need to moderate their feelings, for example, that no one should ever feel extreme anger or love. I concur with Norman[65] who takes the mean to concern the relationship between reason and emotion. As noted, experiencing emotions is an important part of the reality of contemporary nursing practice. Moreover, it is not always simple for nurses to work through their emotions and hit the mean when it comes to exercising the virtues. For example, although a nurse wants to be kind she also realizes that some patients are manipulative; showing too much kindness can then prove counter-productive. Another example concerns the virtue of honesty. If a nurse on a mental health ward was *always completely* honest, this might create difficult situations for other nurses on the ward. Suppose a patient asks an 'honest' nurse about the side effects of a medication and this nurse replies with a long list of relevant side effects. But on another occasion, a different nurse responds to the same question by not revealing some of the side effects; this second nurse responds in this manner because he does not wish to deter the patient from taking the medication as it is having beneficent effects.[66] Finding the mean involves the use of judgement and moral wisdom especially, I think, moral perception. Moral perception helps the nurse to see and discern meaning in a wide range of morally relevant features; clinical information will be taken into account as well as other relevant pieces of information that apply to the specific situation. In brief, moral perception helps to identify and clarify the morally relevant features of morally complex situations. The virtue-based approach to morality can be accused of setting extremely high standards of behaviour for nurses. I accept that it is not always easy to be virtuous; indeed for perhaps the majority of people, cultivating the virtues will be an extremely difficult, though not impossible, endeavour. However, my conception of the virtue-based approach does not claim that nurses must always be virtuous, i.e., it does not follow that the virtue-based nurse should always be, for example, courageous. There will be many times when these virtues are exercised. It is, however, also clear that by using moral wisdom a nurse will make a decision based on the morally (and clinically) relevant features of each specific situation. For example, regarding the virtue of courage, a patient is demanding risky cardiac surgery, which the patient's wife and surgeon are unhappy about; indeed the latter decides not to attempt the surgery. By using moral wisdom, the nurse judges that she would be acting badly, for example, foolishly or naively, if she acted as an advocate for the patient on this occasion. The nurse makes a judgement that the surgeon is acting well, e.g., he is acting from the virtues of honesty, benevolence and non-malevolence. The nurse (and surgeon) decides that going ahead with the operation would be reckless; they also judge that the patient is being selfish because they believe that he is ignoring his wife's feelings. On this occasion, the nurse concludes that to act as the patient's advocate would be an example of acting badly.

Conflicts between virtues

The above discussion regarding the use of moral wisdom and judgement is relevant in responding to another common criticism of the virtue-based approach to morality. This criticism is that virtues conflict and a person has no way of knowing which virtue to exercise. This claim is often held to be a serious objection towards virtue ethics and the virtue-based approach to morality. I shall make four responses to this criticism. First, I hold that conflicts between virtues should be expected given the moral complexity of human lives. Critics,[67] however, suggest that conflicts between virtues are a serious disadvantage of the virtue-based approach and more specifically, critics allege that the lack of a single rule or a decision procedure is a major flaw of the virtue-based approach. In my view, however, an adequate normative ethics should acknowledge that conflicts between obligations or virtues will arise because of the subjective and value-laden moral complexities of human lives. This is particularly true of nursing practice, which is saturated with innumerable complex moral tensions. My second point is a reiteration of two previous points relating to the claim 'a nurse has no way of knowing which virtue to exercise when two or more virtues conflict'. The first point is that the action-guidance available from thinking about the virtues such as kindness means that a nurse will have a good idea as to what to do. One can first eliminate actions, thoughts and feelings that are unkind, cruel and callous, in other words, examples of acting from the vices. Then, second, the use of moral imagination and reflection on the v-rule 'be kind' can conjure up examples of kind actions, thoughts and feelings. The second related point is that a nurse might prioritize one virtue over another, for example, she might believe that justice is more important than patience in a specific situation. Irrespective of other virtues, the nurse will have an idea regarding what to do and how to be, i.e., in this situation she will act in just ways and think and feel justly. Third, the essential question at the heart of the conflicts problem can be framed: 'How ought a nurse to act in a situation in which she could act from virtue x or virtue y?' Let the virtue of respectfulness be x and justice be y. Return for a moment to the example of Carol the community nurse and Jack, the patient with PD. Although it was perhaps not explicit, in this scenario the virtues of respectfulness and justice were in conflict. The options were: should Carol get Jack out of bed or allow him to have another hour in bed? Carol acted from the virtue of respectfulness; she utilized moral wisdom and judgement in her decision-making. Taking into account the morally (and clinically) relevant features, Carol believed that being respectful and leaving Jack in bed a little longer would help him to fare well. Carol also thought about the virtue of justice and Jack's needs. Based in part on her previous practice, Carol concluded that it would be unfair to insist that Jack should get out of bed; on previous similar occasions, she had respected other patients' views. According to Carol, one of the central questions was 'Why should I insist that Jack should get out of bed when I have allowed other patients to lie in bed longer?' I noted earlier that clinical situations will often require more than one virtue to be exercised. This scenario is an example of this claim because besides being respectful, Carol also acted from kindness in allowing Jack to sleep longer. Another community nurse might have acted from the obligation of non-maleficence; she might have persuaded Jack to get out of bed because she wanted to prevent the development of a sacral pressure sore; in other words she placed a higher moral value on minimizing harms than respecting Jack's wishes. However, I need to make it clear that I am not suggesting that a nurse who acts in accordance with an obligation such as non-maleficence is *unable* to act kindly. Instead, the point is that it can seem so important for some nurses to act from obligations (both moral and legal) that other morally important features are neglected. My last point is that the virtues are excellences of character; admirable and praiseworthy traits that help their possessor and others to lead morally good lives. I understand that making decisions regarding the moral importance of virtues is problematic especially for people who are drawn to the certainty provided by empiricism. However, the choice is between two (or more) virtues; thus by definition subsequent actions, thoughts and feelings will be morally good and exert a positive impact on patients' lives. Acting from the virtues of, for example, justice or kindness will, in different ways, help the patient to fare well. The actions, thoughts and feelings that spring from both virtues will be different but, each in their own way will contribute towards the patient faring well during and beyond illness.

Conclusions

Traditional accounts of consequentialism and deontology neglect the crucial role played by judgement and moral wisdom in the moral lives of nurses and patients; indeed, act-consequentialism with its single rule – maximize best consequences – holds that the use of judgement is a sign of a defective moral person.[68] I have shown how the virtue-based approach to morality takes these phenomena seriously; indeed, they lie at the heart of this approach. I have characterized the three features of the virtue-based approach to moral decision-making in nursing practice: (1) the exercise of moral virtues; (2) the use of judgement; and (3) the use of moral wisdom. As noted, certain forms of the deontic approach pay homage to (1), but traditional accounts ignore and deride the use of (2) and (3). However, as with all moral theories, several notable problems afflict the virtue-based approach to morality. I have tried to respond to these problems in particular the 'conflicts between virtues' problem. I believe that my responses provide an adequate defence of the virtue-based approach to morality in contemporary nursing practice. The virtues and virtue ethics have numerous merits, which were identified in Chapters 3 and 5. Within the context of nursing practice, merits of the virtue-based approach include:

- Nurses utilize the language of the virtues in clinical practice;
- Adequate action-guidance is provided through rigorous thinking about the v-rules and the virtue and vice terms
- The role played by emotions in the moral lives of patients and nurses is taken seriously;
- Empowerment and patient-centred care are promoted;
- The use of judgement and moral wisdom is recognized as being very important for nurses.

My conception of the virtue-based approach to morality has distinct advantages for contemporary nurses compared to the traditional obligation-based theories of consequentialism and deontology. A strong version of virtue ethics, one that provides adequate action-guidance for nurses is a viable possibility. Therefore, my major conclusion is that an action-guiding version of the virtue-based approach to morality and moral decision-making is a convincing and plausible alternative to the traditional and inadequate accounts of consequentialism and deontology that are more commonly invoked within nursing practice.

9
MacIntyre's Account of the Virtues

Introduction

I have argued that an action-guiding version of the virtue-based approach to morality is plausible, much more so than many critics suggest. I believe that this approach offers many advantages compared with the traditional accounts of consequentialism and deontology that are currently predominant within contemporary nursing practice and the field of nursing ethics. While I believe that my account of the virtue-based approach is reasonably convincing, I aim to strengthen it a little further. Therefore, in this chapter I will examine MacIntyre's work on virtue ethics because his ideas on the virtues provide my account with a more rigorous philosophical foundation.

MacIntyre is dissatisfied with and pessimistic about many of the claims inherent in modernism. The objects of his disapproval include some of the claims made by contemporary political philosophy in particular liberalism and modern moral philosophy especially what he terms the 'Enlightenment project'. What does MacIntyre propose as an alternative moral theory?[1] In brief, he responds by proposing a neo-Aristotelian ethics that is (a) teleological, (b) socially contextualized and (c) historicized. According to MacIntyre, these three features are not found in contemporary obligation-based moral theories; or, if these features are present they are given low priority. I shall examine MacIntyre's concerns with contemporary ethics in more detail because this provides the philosophical background and motivation for his moral theory. Then I shall present the three major theses defended in *After Virtue* that constitute his account of the virtues. I end this chapter by considering some of the objections and merits of MacIntyre's theory.

MacIntyre on modern moral philosophy

MacIntyre's dismissive claims about modern moral philosophy are similar in some respects to the rejection of Kantianism and utilitarianism that Anscombe[2] made in 1958. While Anscombe's thesis was grounded in the lack of a theistic deity in contemporary society, one can see in her writings the seeds of MacIntyre's ideas. (Indeed, Anscombe has influenced several philosophers who might be labelled 'anti-theorists', besides MacIntyre another example is Williams.[3]) Prior to *After Virtue*, MacIntyre began to demonstrate his disagreement with and dislike of the substance of modern moral philosophy.[4] In short, he criticized the theories and the theorists because the former were not socially and historically contextualized, i.e., they tended to ignore the important role played by history and social theory in moral philosophy. The result was that the development of moral theories and moral agents over time, place and culture was ignored. Furthermore, the historical context of the philosophers who advanced such theories and ideas was also neglected. In *After* Virtue, MacIntyre continues to develop these claims. Additionally, he is disgruntled with modern moral philosophy because it is predominantly concerned with trying to resolve intractable moral disagreements including irresolvable dilemmas. One reason why such dilemmas are irresolvable is that conflicting moral positions invoke incommensurable premises, for example, the ethics of abortion invokes moral rights and the Kantian idea of universalizability. However, the meanings now given to these (and other) moral notions are hidden, disjointed or empty of substance, i.e., they are meaningless. This is principally because the meaning of these moral notions derived originally from historical contexts far different from contemporary modernism. One of MacIntyre's major claims is that some of the social and political arrangements typical of modernity prove hostile to the cultivation of the virtues. MacIntyre argues that the virtues can only flourish if one has an adequate, shared idea of what the good life for man is and for him, modernism ignores this Aristotelian concept. MacIntyre argues that in contemporary Western cultures, virtue terms such as 'justice' and 'desert' are used out of context. These terms have been redefined to refer to obligations to obey the moral rules or principles of justice. MacIntyre argues that this flawed view of the virtues is adopted by modernism especially contemporary liberalism. Consequently liberalism fails to develop a shared view of the virtues. Moreover because liberalism is wrought up in the idea of the capitalist market, the vices of, for example, individualism and acquisitiveness are cultivated instead. Finally, liberalism or more specifically liberal theory is also committed to an impartial and neutral view of the good; it maintains an unbiased view between competing conceptions of the good. One result of this is that the virtues in particular justice, honesty and courage are not cultivated.

I shall now describe MacIntyre's argument, although I limit this discussion to the MacIntyre found in *After Virtue* and specifically, to the three major theses presented in Chapters 14 and 15 in which MacIntyre develops his account of the virtues. I shall describe his argument in three sections (S1–S3):

- S1 – The role and importance of MacIntyre's narrative conception of the self in morality;
- S2 – MacIntyre on practices, goods and the virtues;
- S3 – The role and importance of a tradition of enquiry in morality.

S1 – The role and importance of MacIntyre's narrative conception of the self in morality

MacIntyre objects to the conception of the 'self' advanced by contemporary liberalism, which views individuals as essentially deciding and choosing beings. He rejects the liberal view that choosing and deciding largely determine the moral worth and value ascribed to an act or person. The liberal self understands the good as only one part of making choices and decisions and this 'self' is the sole arbiter of decision-making. This conception of the self can say, for example, 'I am what I decide to be' or 'I shall choose x over y'; it can, if it so desires, include or ignore any or all of the contingent social features of one's existence. Against this conception of the self, MacIntyre proposes a narrative conception. In *After Virtue* MacIntyre writes:

> Man is in his actions and practice, as well as in his fictions, essentially a story-telling animal. He is not essentially, but becomes through his history, a teller of stories that aspire to truth. But the key question for men is not about their own authorship; I can only answer the question 'What am I to do?' if I can answer the prior question 'of what story or stories do I find myself a part?' We enter human society, that is, with one or more imputed characters – roles into which we have been drafted – and we have to learn what they are in order to be able to understand how others respond to us and how our responses to them are apt to be construed.[5]

It is clear that MacIntyre rejects the liberal idea that an individual is principally a decider and chooser. According to MacIntyre, a person has an identity that is partly conceived before he or she makes any decisions or choices. Therefore, the central question in agents' moral lives is not concerned with decisions and choices, which we ought to make 'but rather [it is] a question about how we are to understand who we are'.[6] I will summarize these two different conceptions of the self. First, liberalism places the emphasis on the idea that humans are primarily choosing and deciding beings. Second, MacIntyre's narrative conception focuses on the moral context, history and background circumstances, which are unchosen but which help to inform and make one's choices meaningful and comprehensible. Why does MacIntyre refer to his view as 'narrative'? Clearly this relates to his claims about man as a story-telling creature. Furthermore, Horton and Mendus hold that MacIntyre's conception of the self is called narrative because

> it implies that answers to questions about what we ought to do involve not merely (or primarily) choosing what to do as individuals, but also, and essentially, discovering who we are in relation to others.[7]

Thus, an important theme is developing, namely, that it is crucial that one reflects on and comprehends how one responds to others and how others respond to us. This thesis about the narrative conception of the self in MacIntyre's moral theory contains both epistemological and normative dimensions. Broadly, for individuals to be properly understood – for one to fully understand oneself – reference to the wider community, to other beings, needs to take place. There is a requirement to understand that one's being is partly constituted through social relations and interpersonal responses. The normative dimension follows from these epistemological claims because these claims have implications for how humans ought to live. This relationship – between the epistemological and normative – is philosophically interesting and stimulating. It is, however, problematic as some critics argue that the normative dimension does not necessarily follow from the epistemological (I discuss this point further in the 'Criticisms' section).

What ought I to do? This pivotal question in moral philosophy lies at the core of obligation-based moral theories. MacIntyre argues that one must acknowledge the importance of the narrative structure of one's life; the story of my life has a certain narrative structure 'in which what I am now is continuous with what I was in the past'.[8] Rather than one's life being principally a set of choices and decisions, it is a *search*, a search for one's own identity, for who or what I am and for what I ought to do.

MacIntyre calls this search a *quest* and it is essential to what he calls 'the unity of a person's life'. On this, he says:

> In what does the unity of an individual life consist? The answer is that its unity is the unity of a narrative embodied in a single life. To ask, 'What is the good for me?' is to ask how best I might live out that unity and bring it to completion. To ask, 'What is the good for man?' is to ask what all answers to the former question must have in common. But now it is important to emphasize that it is the systematic asking of these two questions and the attempt to answer them in deed as well as in word which provides the moral life with its unity. The unity of a human life is the unity of a narrative quest.[9]

The most important part of discovering the unity of one's life lies in asking the questions 'What is the good for me?' and 'What is the good for man?' The unity of one's life is, in part, achieved by aiming to provide responses to these two questions in terms of both one's actions and dialogue. However, it should be noted that this unity to which MacIntyre refers must be understood from within a social context and without this perspective, there can be no substance to a person's life; however, it is notable to remember that according to MacIntyre one cannot choose one's social context.

S2 – MacIntyre on practices, goods and the virtues

MacIntyre objects to the lack of teleology within contemporary liberalism; indeed the latter denies the possibility of a telos for man. One result of this is liberalism's inability to evaluate what and who we are and compare and contrast this with what and who we ought to be. In short, MacIntyre proposes a moral theory that has the virtues at its core. MacIntyre accords social context a prominent role in morality. Furthermore, he thinks that it is crucial for humans to consider how their present identity has been formed from the past; MacIntyre refers to this as the 'given' in our lives. These ideas are also present in his concept of a practice, about which MacIntyre writes:

> By a 'practice' I am going to mean any coherent and complex form of socially established co-operative human activity through which goods internal to that form of activity are realized in the course of trying to achieve those standards of excellence which are appropriate to, and partially definitive of, that form of activity, with the result

that human powers to achieve excellence, and human conceptions of the ends and goods involved, are systematically extended.[10]

Examples of practices given by MacIntyre include chess, football, farming, architecture, music, painting and the enquiries of physics, chemistry, biology and history. One of the most important points about practices, for moral philosophy at least, is that there are standards of excellence internal to each practice. On this Horton and Mendus write:

> For example, in order to play chess well, a player must heed the standards which define the playing of chess. Not just anything counts as playing chess well, and the features which do count are ones which are defined by the practice. They are not matters for individual preference or decision-making.[11]

For MacIntyre, morality in general and the virtues in particular should be viewed as practice-based. Indeed he claims that the concept of a practice is crucial to an adequate and satisfactory account of the virtues. People cannot simply decide and choose what acting morally well means to them; instead acting well is to be determined according to the type of practice(s) one is engaged in. Thus instead of rigid moral obligations, rules and principles the virtues have a central position in MacIntyre's conception of morality, indeed he argues that morality should be conceived as a life that embodies the virtues. One's understanding of why particular character traits count as virtues and indeed on the question of what virtues are, depend upon our ability to (a) recognize the role that virtues play in practices and (b) reflect critically on the central role played by the virtues in the narrative unity of the self. In Chapter 14 of *After Virtue* entitled 'The Nature of the Virtues', MacIntyre provides a tentative definition of a virtue. He writes:

> A virtue is an acquired human quality the possession and exercise of which tends to enable us to achieve those goods which are internal to practices and the lack of which effectively prevents us from achieving any such goods.[12]

MacIntyre holds that only social and political arrangements that sustain the practices and ensure the supply of the internal goods exclusive to each practice are justifiable. Before I provide MacIntyre's revised formulation of a virtue, the idea of internal goods requires some clarification. An obvious question perhaps, but are there external goods? The response to this is affirmative. MacIntyre uses the game of chess to explain the distinction between these two types of goods. It is possible to gain both internal and external goods by playing chess. Examples of external goods include money, status and prestige. These goods can be achieved in other ways besides playing chess; they are only externally and contingently attached to the playing of chess. MacIntyre asserts that the achievement of external goods 'is never to be had *only* by engaging in some particular kind of practice'.[13] Conversely, the goods internal to playing chess – the practice of chess – cannot be achieved by any other means but by playing chess or as MacIntyre adds another game of that kind. What might the internal goods of chess be? While it is difficult to state categorically what these might be they could include the sorts of feelings and attitudes developed and sustained in those who play chess and take pride in aiming to be excellent at playing chess. These goods are achieved through striving for excellence; people aim to improve on previous practitioners whose participation in the practice has formed the history and standards of the practice. Why does MacIntyre call these goods internal? Two reasons are given:

> First, as I have already suggested, because we can only specify them in terms of chess or some other game of that specific kind and by means of examples from such games … and secondly because they can only be identified and recognized by the experience of participating in the practice in question.[14]

What are the internal goods of chess? MacIntyre holds that it is impossible for one who does not play the game of chess to know the answer to this question. For him, people ought to relate their lives to the numerous different types of practices that make up their lives and the virtues are crucial to this process. His reformulated definition of a virtue, which takes this into account suggests virtues are to be understood as dispositions

> which will not only sustain practices and enable us to achieve the goods internal to practices, but which will also sustain us in the relevant kind of quest for the good, by enabling us to overcome the harms, dangers, temptations and distractions which we encounter, and which will furnish us with increasing self-knowledge and increasing knowledge of the good.[15]

It is useful to repeat the four claims made in the above quote. The virtues:

I. Sustain practices;
II. Enable humans to achieve the internal goods of practices;
III. Ensure that we continue on our search or quest for the good life;
IV. Help to provide us with greater self-knowledge and knowledge of the good life for man.

Thus the virtues help us to proceed with our search for the good life. They help us to prevent or deal with harmful aspects of life that may lead us away from the quest for the good. Furthermore, the virtues develop one's knowledge of oneself and knowledge of what the good for one consists in. Before I consider MacIntyre's concept of a tradition, I shall comment further on what MacIntyre means by a good life. As noted in Chapter 3, different virtues are necessary to meet the ends of practices that humans participate in. For example, the virtues required to achieve the ends of law will differ from those needed in farming or nursing. Furthermore, virtues are needed to sustain different types of communities such as political and social communities. Men and women can search for the good in their moral lives, while philosophers can enquire about the nature of the good. MacIntyre provisionally concludes that the good life for man is

> the life spent in seeking for the good life for man, and the virtues necessary for the seeking are those which will enable us to understand what more and less the good life for man is.[16]

However, the view that the good life is the life spent *seeking* the good life is open to criticism (this is discussed in the 'Criticisms' section). For MacIntyre, the practices and the exercise of the virtues that sustain the practices must knit together in such a way that people come to understand that the life of virtue is indeed a good way of living one's life.[17] It should not be assumed that people will *know* that the virtuous life is worthwhile, more so than say an egoistical life. But how one can know that the life of virtue is a good life and how different practices *knit* together are indeed complex questions.

S3 – The role and importance of a tradition of enquiry in morality

To recap: first, MacIntyre has provided a narrative conception of the self that has advantages over liberalism's conception such as, it takes seriously the moral context, history and background circumstances of peoples' lives. Second, MacIntyre has defined the virtues in relation to practices and then linked this to the good life for man. The third (and final) stage of his account of the virtues concerns the concept of a tradition of enquiry. According to MacIntyre, it is important to remember that contemporary liberalism ignores the important role played by social context and history in morality. One result of this is that the given in one's moral life is not acknowledged by liberalism. MacIntyre argues that people cannot search for the good for man or exercise the virtues *qua* individuals. He provides two reasons for this claim. First, people live in different social circumstances and living the good life changes according to these circumstances. For instance, the good life for a 6th-century Athenian general will be quite different to the good life for a 17th-century farmer. Second, people have particular social identities with which they approach their specific circumstances. For example, I am someone's son, my sister is someone's daughter, I am a member of the nursing profession and a citizen of England. MacIntyre believes that what is good for me *must* be the good for others who take on these roles. Furthermore, MacIntyre writes:

> I inherit from the past of my family, my city, my tribe, my nation, a variety of debts, inheritances, rightful expectations and obligations. These constitute the given of my life, my moral starting point. This is in part what gives my life its own moral particularity.[18]

This reference to debts, inheritances, rightful expectations and obligations helps to shed some light on one's understanding of MacIntyre's phrase, the 'given in our lives'. These features of the moral life are inherited – consciously or not – from the past. MacIntyre seems to be suggesting that these features will ensure particular moral starting points. While this implies (at least on the surface) a form of individualism at odds with his previous claims (especially those in S1), it is balanced by his view that part of one's identity consists in social and historical roles. These roles consist in ends that apply to each person who takes on that role. It seems to me that MacIntyre is no liberal when regarding the narrative conception of the self, he says: 'The story of my life is always embedded in the story of those communities from which I derive my identity'.[19] In other words: 'I cannot map my identity and I am unable to keep track of who and what I am without reference to other beings who form the community I live in'. On MacIntyre's view much of what I am is inherited. Parts of the past impinge on my present. I am part of a history although I may not realize this. As such, I am a bearer of a tradition of enquiry. In *After Virtue* MacIntyre defines a living tradition as:

> An historically extended, socially embodied argument, and an argument precisely in part about the goods which constitute that tradition.[20]

Greater clarification on this definition is given by Mulhall and Swift who write:

> A tradition is constituted by a set of practices and is a mode of understanding their importance and worth; it is the medium by which such practices are shaped and transmitted across generations.[21]

Mulhall and Swift state that there are many types of traditions including moral (e.g. humanism), religious (e.g. Catholicism) and economic (e.g. a profession). It is important to note that traditions are not static, but dynamic. Possibilities exist not only for an individual to embark on a quest and to acknowledge the given in one's life, but also to critically reflect on the nature and content of the traditions and practices which one finds oneself a part. This dynamism is described by Horton and Mendus who remark:

> Traditions change and develop over time; some decay and fall into terminal disrepair and some emerge in response to changed circumstances.[22]

Because of this dynamism, MacIntyre believes that the concept of a tradition is not conservative; however, later we shall see that others disagree with him on this. MacIntyre's moral theory can now be understood to encompass (1) a narrative conception of the self, (2) a conception of practices and the crucial role of the virtues in the sustenance of the practices and (3) an understanding of a tradition of enquiry that situates the aforementioned in a wider context. As noted earlier, the diverse sets of practices that exist within society define the virtues. These practices are situated within and help to sustain a tradition of enquiry, 'which provides the resources with which the individual may pursue his or her quest for the good'.[23] Crucial components of this quest are moral deliberation and action, which rely heavily on standards of rationality that form part of the overall tradition of enquiry in question. Since *After Virtue*, MacIntyre has increasingly focused on the notion of rationality and the concept of a tradition.

Criticisms of MacIntyre's thesis

In this section I discuss further some of the detail in MacIntyre's moral argument as outlined in *After Virtue*. I present several criticisms levelled against his theory and again organize these within S1–S3:

- S1 – The role and importance of MacIntyre's narrative conception of the self in morality;
- S2 – MacIntyre on practices, goods and the virtues;
- S3 – The role and importance of a tradition of enquiry in morality.

S1 – The role and importance of MacIntyre's narrative conception of the self in morality

On the epistemological and normative dimensions of the self

MacIntyre alludes to the fact that his narrative conception of the self contains both epistemological and normative dimensions and as noted, Horton and Mendus pick up on this. Consider the following example. John is a 40-year-old farmer married to Jean. They have two children, one son, Daniel aged ten, and a daughter, Julie aged five. John has farmed all his life, inheriting his farm from his parents ten years ago. He employs two aides, Brian and Todd. There are other farms in the surrounding area, the most prominent one is owned by John's friend, Jack. For John to get to know himself well, for him to strive to understand who and what he is, he needs to be aware and understand that his being is partly constituted through his relations with and responses to others including his relationships with Jean, Daniel and Julie. Additionally, there are his relationships with Brian and Todd to consider and how he gets on and responds to Jack, other local farmers and the local community. These claims are epistemological in nature because they deal with beliefs about one's identity (these claims also have a metaphysical component). Horton and Mendus claim that the normative dimension – how one should live one's life – follows from the epistemological claims. In other words, knowing who one is and what kind of person one is and relating this knowledge to getting on with others has implications for how one ought to live. These epistemological and normative claims appear plausible. It is clear that these claims apply to general ethics as a whole and not only to virtue ethics. A person who fails to understand or does not attempt to understand oneself, one who takes little or no interest in how one responds to others (or how others respond to one) could be called egoistic, self-interested or even, in an extreme case, amoral. If everyone acted in self-interested ways, then social relations would crumble or fail to develop in the first place. Because of their lack of concern for others, people would show no interest in cultivating the virtues, so for example, trust, honesty and loyalty would be marginalized. The lack of such virtues would not merely be responsible for the failure of human relationships; business and economics would also suffer badly. As someone who wants to be virtuous, it is important that when I reflect on my thoughts and plan my actions, I take others' interests into account and I would add that I ought to care about others' interests. Suppose that Ethel has just started work as a typist in my small company. I know that one of my positive traits is showing patience with others. This trait did not come naturally; I had to work hard to cultivate it; I observed how being patient helped others and so I aim to be patient with others. Nancy, the senior typist, complains to me that Ethel is 'just too slow'. Nancy believes that Ethel should have a typing speed in excess of 35 wpm. I talk with Ethel and during the conversation it emerges that Ethel, though experienced, is a very nervous person who needs a few weeks to settle into a new post. I tell Ethel that we can wait for her to settle in. I ask Ethel if I can discuss this with Nancy. After gaining her permission, I explain the situation to Nancy and ask that she is more patient with Ethel. Two weeks later, Ethel has settled into her new job and has made a few friends. She now types at 60 wpm. This example illustrates the moral value and worth of perceiving one's positive and negative character traits and caring about and wherever possible helping others. It seems to me that epistemological and normative claims and the necessary link between them, forms the basis of morality.

On choosing and deciding

If one accepts MacIntyre's primary claim that contemporary liberalism views people as *essentially* choosing and deciding beings, then the secondary claim, that the process of deciding and choosing determines the moral worth of a person or a person's acts, remains open to criticism because there is more to this than *merely* choosing and deciding. Perhaps the majority of liberals are deontologists who instruct us to act in accordance with moral obligations, for example, beneficence, justice and respect for autonomy. Other liberals are consequentialists, concerned with maximizing or optimizing good consequences. As noted in

Chapter 4, deontologists and consequentialists focus on actions and especially on the question 'What should I do?' Their response is to invoke moral obligations, rules and principles, while deontologists also invoke the notion of moral rights. The latter theorists are convinced that the moral value of an act concerns not only the aforementioned moral notions, but also moral concepts such as intention. While I accept that one needs to choose which of the aforementioned moral notions will guide one's actions, I have also noted that morality includes other relevant features. And although exercising judgement involves a series of choices and decisions this phenomenon and also moral wisdom require extensive examination. MacIntyre is sceptical of the prime role liberals assign to choosing and deciding. MacIntyre's claim that one is 'drafted' into human roles that provide one with one's character suggests that he has anti-liberal tendencies, because the use of 'drafted' implies one has no choice. This lends some support to the idea that in wanting a moral theory that takes into account the role of history and society, MacIntyre has gone overboard in his criticism of the idea of 'choosing and deciding'. His theory appears to be severely anti-liberal and it does not need to be.

On the good life

According to MacIntyre, men and women can search for the good in their moral lives. For him, it is *searching* for the good life that actually constitutes a good life. Two points here are worth making. First, there is no mention of a shared conception of the good. But if each person can search and discover a good, then this is a liberal and not a MacIntyrian idea. Second and more importantly, how would MacIntyre respond to the following: 'During one's search for the good life, on several occasions one displays certain vices for instance impatience and intolerance; is this an example of a good life?' It is difficult to imagine what MacIntyre's strategy could be here. I doubt he would conclude that this sort of life is a life of vice because acting from the vices 'on several occasions' does not constitute *a life* of vice. Indeed it suggests that there were many times when one did not act from the virtues. MacIntyre claims that the virtues necessary to search for the good life are those that help shed light on what the good life is. These virtues are intellectual virtues that were noted by Aristotle in Chapter 3. Wisdom, both theoretical and practical, is an example of an intellectual virtue. The role of wisdom is quite obvious when one is searching for something, i.e., it is beneficial to the searcher if one possesses wisdom rather than a caring virtue such as compassion.

Denying a telos for man?

Another example of MacIntyre's characterization of liberalism is his implication that it denies a telos for man. Is a telos for man the *only* way in which one can formulate who one ought to be and what one ought to do? If these two claims are correct, then it is true to suggest that liberalism is unable to contrast who one is and what one does with who one ought to be and what one ought to do. A simple yet accurate characterization of liberalism holds that each person is a choosing and deciding being. If correct, this then explains why a telos for man is denied by it. In his defence, MacIntyre does suggest that human choices are important to our 'selves'. However, on his view one is required to take other features into account, for example, moral context, history and background circumstances because these features help us to understand our choices and decisions. I concur with MacIntyre on this. Without these features, our choices and decisions would be effectively meaningless. On MacIntyre's view, one could conclude that liberals regard choosing and deciding as sufficient in morality. MacIntyre believes, however, that choosing and deciding are only necessary in morality and are only of use when contextualized. However, some liberals would agree with MacIntyre on this. Therefore, MacIntyre has done contemporary liberalism a disservice by inaccurately representing it in particular the liberal conception of the self.

Man as a story-telling animal

MacIntyre says that man is *essentially* a story-telling animal. Is this accurate? During childhood in particular, stories and story-telling are undeniably an important part of one's moral education. As exemplified by so-called fairy tales, often such stories do not aim at the truth. But they serve a vital role in entertaining and amusing children; moreover they teach children about good and bad people, the world and one's place in it. In adulthood too, stories do not always aim at the truth. For example, some types of stories, riddles for example, aim to stretch our imagination, jokes aim to make us laugh and historical stories aim to tell us what and why events occurred in the past. The latter kinds of stories are an example of narratives that aim at the truth or at least the historian's version of the truth. Much of MacIntyre's claim of course depends upon what is meant by the 'truth'; several theories of truth are described in the philosophical literature, for example, coherence[24] and pragmatic[25] theories of truth. It will in part depend upon which theory is adopted as to whether the telling of stories is *always* a means of relaying truthful information. MacIntyre's narrative conception of the self is relevant to moral philosophy; if by 'stories' he means not just fairy tales but also the relaying of information about one's life to other people, then I would agree that man is *essentially* a story-telling animal.

S2 – MacIntyre on practices, goods and the virtues

The flourishing of the virtues in modernity

MacIntyre argues that the virtues cannot flourish within modernity because radical disagreement exists on the notion of the good life for man. His conclusion is that the virtues will therefore be marginalized. On this claim, Mason asks:

> Why does it follow that the virtues must suffer when there is no agreement on a substantive conception of the good.[26]

To illustrate MacIntyre's argument, Mason focuses on distributive justice. To summarize MacIntyre: justice as a virtue was originally conceived in terms of desert. What one deserved was judged according to one's contribution to the community, which held a shared conception of the good. However, as noted earlier, the virtue of justice has become redefined in terms of a disposition to obey the rules and principles of justice. In part, this has happened because of the lack of any consensus regarding what forms the community's good. But because there are different rules and principles of justice, there is radical disagreement on the nature and content of justice as a virtue (if it is viewed as a virtue at all). Mason is uncertain about what MacIntyre's precise point is. He believes that MacIntyre might be making one of three points. First, the virtue of justice will be marginalized because it is understood as supplementary to the rules and principles of justice. However, even in this context, Mason claims that justice as a virtue could still thrive. He argues that there is no reason why the status of justice within our culture *must* diminish despite the fact that various conceptions of justice as a virtue exist. He concludes that virtue terms – desert, for instance – could remain widely used in everyday discourse and people could continue to highly value the virtues. Second, the virtue of justice – understood according to MacIntyre as a trait needed to sustain a particular practice – will be marginalized. Mason thinks that justice as a virtue includes one's ability to impartially judge one's contribution to the community's good. Therefore, if the virtue of justice was understood as a disposition to obey the rules and principles of justice, it might be conceived as a disposition to obey the rule 'people should be rewarded in accordance with their contribution to the community's good'.[27] Mason believes that this rule is plausible although he is aware that MacIntyre's response might be to argue that this rule would still be insufficient because there would still be no shared conception of the good. Mason believes that this reply would lead MacIntyre into a tautology. Mason writes:

> Justice, conceived (at least in part) as a disposition to reward people according to what they deserve on the basis of their contribution to the good of the community will not flourish where there is radical disagreement, since part of what it is for it to flourish is for people to share a conception of the community's good and to believe that contributions to it should be rewarded.[28]

The third possible point is that MacIntyre might be saying that justice, as a virtue needed to sustain practices, cannot flourish unless this conception is widely accepted. This is because if there is no practice-based conception of the virtues, then the shared practices that ground and define the virtues will not survive. This idea links to MacIntyre's claim that individuals are unable to seek the good life or exercise the virtues only *qua* individuals. The point here is that some form of shared understanding about the practices and their internal goods is required to sustain the practice in question. And the follow up claim is that if consensus is reached, then a measure of cooperation will be too. Mutual cooperation includes forming and maintaining good relationships between individuals helped through the cultivation of the virtues. However, Mason counters this argument by suggesting that while it avoids the aforementioned tautology, he believes that for the virtues to flourish there does not need to be a shared conception of the good, and the virtues need not be the same across communities. On the flourishing of the virtues, Mason writes:

> The virtues might also flourish in a society made up of a number of different practices, each practice involving a group of individuals who shared a conception of the good, and hence who could co-operate with each other in pursuit of it.[29]

I accept this claim. Justice as a virtue is distinct from justice as a disposition to obey the principle of justice. As noted previously, the difference is partly a matter of moral motivation. That is, the virtue of justice is a character trait that individuals cultivate and exercise on a habitual basis. They do so because they think it is valuable for its own sake and because they understand that being just will help to benefit others.

Acting from the obligation of justice is different because one can act in accordance with moral obligations, rules and principles without accepting and understanding what it means to think and feel just. The obligation or principle of justice focuses on just actions and the motive is deontic. However as long as individuals value the content of justice as a virtue (and other virtues too), a real sense of moral admiration for those who are just, and a dedicated and consistent attempt to foster the virtues then it seems to me that the virtues can flourish. Moreover, I agree with Mason on three points. First, there does not need to be a shared conception of the good. Second, the virtues need not be the same across communities and third, the virtues can flourish in different types of practices where within each practice a shared conception of the good exists. MacIntyre suggests several times in *After Virtue* that he might agree with the third point insofar as he readily accepts that different types of practices exist in society. I doubt whether MacIntyre would insist that there ought to be just one shared conception of the good within all of these practices. Even given the third point, I would expect some people within a specific practice not to entirely agree on the conception of the good. There would probably be some shared items on each person's list; debate could centre on which of these items are most plausible and why. Moreover, there need not be any utilitarian calculus performed. Furthermore, complete consensus on the good among many individuals is something that is unrealistic and not worthy of admiration. As Rawls[30] remarks, disagreement over different conceptions of the good is to be expected in a modern democratic society. MacIntyre responds to these comments by arguing that such disagreements are resolvable but only by appealing to a form of Thomism, a tradition of moral thought based upon the work of Thomas Aquinas. Crudely, he thinks that his version of Thomism has rationally compelling reasons that will convince others to jettison their own theories and adopt Thomism instead. In *Whose Justice? Which Rationality?*,[31] MacIntyre's explores his version of Thomism and unsurprisingly, he adopts a fixed conception of the good for man which ensures there are no radical disagreements in morality and politics. MacIntyre aims to show in *Whose Justice? Which Rationality?* why other theorists should abandon their traditions of moral thought. He insists that once they understand his version of Thomism, they will indeed do so.

On practices

The virtues are not merely required to engage in the practices, nor are they just required to meet the ends of each practice in a morally (and technically) excellent manner. Instead the practices *define* what the virtues are. In other words, the practices tell us which traits are to be counted as virtues and why, and provides their content.

Miller on MacIntyre's notion of a practice

Miller[32] makes an important distinction between what he calls self-contained and purposive practices. He accuses MacIntyre of missing this important distinction. Miller believes that this distinction has implications for how the virtues – most notably, courage and justice – are understood and how they relate to the internal goods. Miller claims that Macintyre's list of practices is so diverse that the notion of a practice is made more complicated than it should be. According to Miller, self-contained practices – for instance, chess and cricket – are entirely concerned with 'the internal goods achieved by participants and the contemplation of these achievements by others'.[33] Conversely, Miller believes that purposive practices serve other (usually) social ends. Miller thinks that MacIntyre's distinction between internal and external goods is well made. However this is because MacIntyre focuses on games such as chess where the distinction is quite obvious. Miller explains that the internal goods gained through playing a fine innings of cricket would be 'incomprehensible in the absence of the game itself'. Miller then claims that 'the standard of excellence involved ... can only be identified by reference to the history of the game'.[34] In other words, the sorts of things – particular skills, strokes, positioning of the bat and so on – that make an innings 'fine' have been developed through the history of the game by previous cricketers. One important point is that self-contained practices can only be judged by those who participate in them. MacIntyre's claim that non-participants have insufficient knowledge to identify the internal goods seems to be excessively exclusive. Miller continues by claiming that in the purposive practices of farming or the activities of physicists or historians, there is an external social purpose that helps to provide the *raison d'etre* of the particular practice. For instance, the social purpose of farming could be understood as 'producing food for the community', while for physicists it might be 'discovering and finding evidence to support the truths of physics'. Judgement on the standards of excellence within these practices can legitimately be made from people who do not participate in the practice. Miller's distinction makes MacIntyre's claims about the differences between the internal and external goods less convincing. For example, in farming there is still the distinction between being an excellent farmer and the various extrinsic goods such as developing a good local reputation and financial reward that might accompany success as a farmer. But on Miller's view because farming has an important social purpose, being an excellent farmer also concerns things that are external to that practice. Miller illustrates his concern by referring to the example of medicine (which MacIntyre mentions in *After Virtue*, but fails to develop). Actually stating what the internal goods of medicine are is not particularly straightforward. Perhaps it is 'being an excellent doctor'. However, Miller points out that this might mean different things. For instance, it could refer to 'someone who is excellent at healing the sick' or to 'someone who carries out the standards of the medical community in an excellent manner'. These two meanings might indeed diverge to a degree. If so, Miller argues that the practice will have fallen victim to professional deformation; he writes: 'A good practice here is one whose standards of excellence are related directly to its wider purpose'.[35]

In self-contained practices such as chess or cricket, the rules and standards can only be assessed internally by practitioners taking part. Whereas with purposive practices, for example, farming, architecture or physics, the practice as a whole can be reviewed by comparing it against the end it is meant to serve. Take medicine as an example. It is possible to compare different forms of medicine, for instance, Chinese versus Western. Or it is possible to compare different forms of surgical techniques, for example, hip replacement operations. Standards of excellence relating to these forms of medicine or techniques may change and these changes may be made following a review of such comparisons. Adopting Miller's distinction between self-contained and purposive practices means that in purposive practices, the standards of excellence and internal goods will be related to the particular ends of the practice. Miller believes that MacIntyre makes a mistake in assuming that all practices are the self-contained type (even farming, which seems to have a clear social worth). Miller believes that this assumption is supported by MacIntyre's examples and by MacIntyre's claim that the standards of excellence are only developed through internal debate with specific practices. This assumption helps to make possible MacIntyre's account of the virtues. For MacIntyre, the virtues are dispositions or traits of character required to sustain the practices and achieve the goods internal to each practice. These goods may alter as practices develop. But newly suggested traits cannot simply qualify as virtues on the basis of some social goal or purpose. However Miller argues that the virtues should be understood as dispositions that sustain purposive practices. Thus any 'list' of virtues must be formulated according to the social goals, ends and purposes that each practice is meant to serve. It follows from this that the virtues themselves are no longer independent or self-sufficient dispositions. Instead they are dependent upon an understanding of a particular society's dominant purposes and needs. According to Miller, the main arena for the manifestation of the virtues will be related to purposive practices – for instance, farming and medicine – and not towards self-contained practices. Miller looks at two specific virtues: courage and justice. He asks 'When do we think of people displaying courage? He has three responses: first, during wartime or on the battlefield; second, when acting humanely in dangerous situations and third when putting up with intense pain with equanimity. He believes these are central cases. One could also speak of courage as that quality displayed by, for instance, parachutists. But here he believes that the term 'daring' is preferable because this activity and others like it are optional, i.e., people participate through choice. For Miller, a distinctly 'moral' term like courage does not appear to be warranted in these lesser cases. On this point, he writes:

> Unlike courage displayed in the service of a valued end such as the saving of life or the defence of one's homeland, courage displayed merely for its own sake is hardly the genuine thing.[36]

Miller's conclusion is that plausible accounts of courage, justice and perhaps other virtues need to relate to purposive, not self-contained, practices. How does MacIntyre respond to Miller's criticisms? In short, MacIntyre rejects these objections; he believes that if practices were valued for their external purposes, then these activities would be hostile or opposed to practices. According to MacIntyre, these types of activities are linked to modern economic systems, which are organized in ways that exclude the necessary features of practices. MacIntyre also charges Miller with missing a crucial distinction 'that between a practice and the way in which it is institutionalized'.[37] This distinction helps one to comprehend (a) how external and internal goods are related and (b) how the virtues relate to internal goods. MacIntyre admits that if in *After Virtue* he had focused in greater detail on productive crafts, for example, fishing and farming, then this distinction and the above two points might have been better realized. He explains this point when he writes:

> The aim internal to such productive crafts, when they are in good order, is never only to catch fish...It is to do so in a manner consonant with the excellences of the craft, so that not only is there a good product, but the craft person is perfected through and in her or his activity.[38]

S3 – The role and importance of a tradition of enquiry in morality

The threat of moral relativism

One of the reoccurring criticisms levelled at MacIntyre's moral theory, as outlined in *After Virtue*, concerns the concept of a tradition. Briefly, the objection is that because his moral theory focuses to such an extent on the idea of a tradition, it collapses into a form of moral relativism. More precisely, the claim is that individuals find themselves trapped within a particular tradition. Because they lack the necessary intellectual and practical resources, they are unable to enter into dialogue and adjudicate between other traditions. The result is that individuals cannot free themselves from the tradition they find themselves in. MacIntyre fails to deal with this objection in *After Virtue*. However he picks up on it in *Whose Justice? Which Rationality?* and *Three Rival Versions of Moral Enquiry*. It is pertinent to note that MacIntyre rejects this objection. Despite morality being essentially tradition-dependent and although the given in peoples' lives derives from traditions, MacIntyre believes that people are able to enter into debate and rational argument between contrasting traditions; therefore in his view moral relativism is avoided.

On liberalism ignoring social and historical contexts in moral philosophy

There may be some truth in MacIntyre's assertion that contemporary liberalism ignores the role of social and historical contexts in moral philosophy. However it does not necessarily follow that because of this, liberalism completely fails to acknowledge the given – what is already present in one's life, through one's past, community and nation – in one's moral life. MacIntyre's characterization of contemporary liberalism is crude. Perhaps I misunderstand MacIntyre, but he appears to confuse two points in his discussion of social roles and identities. First, he believes that all individuals have particular social identities; I have no dispute with this claim. This means that people all have individual identities. Second, MacIntyre claims that the good for one person *must* be the good for others who take on that role. The use of 'must' here is rigid and deontic in terms of motive. More notable, however, is the fact that MacIntyre appears to confuse social roles with one's particular character and there are grounds for believing that these are distinct. For example, it does not necessarily follow that Jack (the son of John) will share the same conception of the good as Brian (the son of Norman). Or that Bruce, a farmer, will share the same conception of the good as Frank, another farmer. These people might hold conceptions of the good that converge at least to some degree. This phenomenon, however, might arise out of coincidence, experience (for example, knowledge of what is needed to be a successful farmer) or sheer luck. Examples of shared items for the good life include good health, sufficient money to live well, good, long-lasting relationships with friends and enjoyable and stimulating jobs. Many people would include some (or all) of these items on their list of goods. But the many different particulars that make ones' lives unique – one's hopes, attitudes, fears and beliefs, not to mention the various pragmatic circumstances that shape human lives – ensure that many of us will conceive of the good life in different ways. (Later in *After Virtue*, MacIntyre says that the given in each of our lives gives us a different moral identity or particularity. Here, he seems to be acknowledging the uniqueness of individuals' lives.)

Conclusions

MacIntyre's account of the virtues has been examined. I have interpreted his account in the form of three sections: the role and importance of a narrative conception of the self in morality; the meaning and nature of practices, goods and the virtues; and the role and importance of a tradition of enquiry in morality. MacIntyre believes that moral philosophers have failed to socially and historically contextualize modern obligation-based moral theories. Such theorists have tended to ignore the important role played by history and social theory in moral philosophy. Instead of a liberal conception of the self, which contemporary liberal theory proposes, MacIntyre advances a narrative conception of the self. The latter conception focuses on the moral context, history and background circumstances of peoples' lives. These are unchosen but help to inform and make one's choices meaningful and comprehensible. According to MacIntyre, man is essentially a story-telling animal. I have provided MacIntyre's conception of a practice. A 'practice' is the name given to a complex series of human activities that strive towards standards of excellence and realize entities called internal goods. MacIntyre's examples of practices include chess and farming. For MacIntyre, a virtue is a disposition that:

- Sustains practices;
- Enables humans to achieve the internal goods of practices;
- Ensures that humans continue on their search or quest for the good life;
- Helps to provide humans with greater self-knowledge and knowledge of the good life for man.

It is difficult to identify the internal goods of a practice; MacIntyre believes that only those people who participate in the practice will be able to do this. The internal goods of chess include the sorts of feelings and attitudes developed and sustained in those who play chess and take pride in aiming to be excellent at playing chess. Conversely, external goods include things such as wealth, power and prestige that can all be obtained by participating in other activities. A tradition of enquiry contextualizes and situates the narrative conception of the self, the practices and the virtues. A tradition can be seen as an intellectual argument that provides a way of understanding the value of practices. Traditions are dynamic and change over time; they shape practices and help them to live on through future generations. Practices are situated within and help to sustain a tradition of enquiry.

I have examined several objections levelled against MacIntyre's account. Perhaps the most notable is Miller's distinction between self-contained and purposive practices. Miller believes that purposive practices such as medicine serve social ends. Self-contained practices such as chess and cricket are entirely concerned with the internal goods of that practice and how participants can achieve the internal goods. It should be clear by now that I share many of MacIntyre's concerns with modern moral philosophy. While it is possible to critique MacIntyre's account of the virtues, it remains rigorous and thought provoking. I believe that some of his ideas are of value and could be applied to nursing ethics and specifically, moral decision-making. Therefore, in the next chapter I will apply some of his key ideas to my conception of the virtue-based approach to morality in nursing practice.

10
MacIntyre's Account of the Virtues and the Virtue-Based Approach to Moral Decision-Making in Nursing Practice

Introduction

Having examined MacIntyre's account of the virtues, it is clear that some of his ideas, for example, those regarding the narrative account of the self and the conception of a practice could be applied to moral decision-making in nursing practice. Therefore, this is what I shall do in this chapter.

Nursing practice, narratives and morality

In Chapter 2, I examined some common emotions that people feel during illness and I noted that the process of hospitalization often intensifies such emotions. I focused on the emotions of anxiety, fear, powerlessness, vulnerability and dependence on others for help. Patients can express their feelings about illness in the form of a narrative. Partly because the emphasis is not solely upon the nature and consequences of actions, the virtue-based approach to morality encourages nurses to listen to patients' narratives. The emphasis in the virtue-based approach is on nurses' and patients' character traits and this approach recognizes the important role played by emotions in the moral life of patients and nurses. Of central importance to the virtue-based approach is the need for nurses to cultivate and exercise moral virtues; the broad aim being to develop and maintain morally excellent care. It seems to me that MacIntyre's narrative conception of the self acknowledges the importance of morally good interpersonal responses. For MacIntyre, the central question in one's moral life is 'How am I to understand who I am?' Thus, questions concerning personal identity and reflection on both intrapersonal and interpersonal responses are crucial features of the moral life; who and what I am concerns context and one's role as a nurse. In Chapter 2, I noted the empowering effects created by listening to patients' narratives. An important feature of the virtue-based nurse is her authentic desire to understand the patient's lived experience of illness. Take a patient with CRA as an example. The virtue-based nurse is motivated to discover how the CRA affects the patient's life, how inflamed joints affect the activities of living and the sorts of problems of living caused by the CRA. The nurse will assimilate information regarding the patient's physical and non-physical interests and needs and here, the virtue of patience will be exercised because this objective is difficult and time-consuming. Virtue-based nurses are motivated to spend time with patients, asking questions and listening to their responses. As noted previously, exercising the moral virtues is admirable and deserves praise precisely because cultivating virtue is arduous and it is easier *not* to be virtuous. Being virtuous requires a serious and sincere commitment to nursing and a dedication to the role of being a morally good nurse. The virtue-based nurse wishes to understand the patient's narrative and she aims to situate the patient at the centre of care; indeed it seems to me that 'patient-centred' care will be more completely addressed if nurses acted from the virtues rather than obligation. Through self-reflection and reflection on the patient's interests and needs, the virtue-based nurse is motivated to ask questions such as 'How in this situation can I help my patient?' and 'How in this situation should I respond to my patient's needs?'

Understanding the narrative conception of the self should help nurses to reflect on patients' pasts, presents and futures. Listening to and understanding a patient's narrative account of illness should steer the nurse to view a patient's time on a hospital ward as only one moment out of that person's entire life. For instance, a nurse is caring for a patient with CRA named John; the 'present' is John's time spent on the ward. But John is 65 years old; he has a 'past', which the nurse knows little about. Granted, some factual information is written in the medical and nursing documentation, but there is no sense of John as a person, no sense of his values, beliefs and life plans. Clearly, no one knows what will happen to John in his 'future'; once he has been discharged, no one knows what will happen to him. MacIntyre's account of morality is context dependent; it is a particularist approach rather than the universal approach adopted by traditional accounts of consequentialism and deontology in particular Kantianism. MacIntyre's account focuses on the moral context, history and background circumstances of one's life, which provides meaning and facilitates an understanding of one's possible decisions, choices, actions and ways of responding to others. Thinking about this wide range of morally relevant features will help nurses to contextualize the patient's unique situation. Naturally, being there does not guarantee that the nurse will see the morally relevant features; this will depend in part on moral wisdom, in particular moral perception.

In response to the question 'What ought I to do?' a nurse can search for her identity by asking questions such as 'Who am I?' According to MacIntyre, one goes on a quest for the unity of one's life and such a quest requires a social context. Important questions that ought to be posed include 'What is the good for me as an individual nurse?', 'What is the good for this team of nurses?' and 'What is the good for my patient in this situation?' According to Horton and Mendus[1] although answers to 'What ought we to do?' involve asking what one should do as an individual, they concern more importantly discovering who one is in relation to other people. Who am I in relation to other nurses? Who am I in relation to my patient? My patient knows me as a nurse, but am I a distant professional, a friend or someone who exercises the virtue of friendliness? In response to these sorts of questions, at least two things are required: reflection (including self-reflection) and self-awareness. As a requirement of moral wisdom, the virtue-based approach advocates the use of reflection; on oneself, other people and the world one inhabits. Does self-reflection promote self-awareness? I believe it helps. Developing self-awareness is crucial to the success of the virtue-based approach; an awareness of one's good and bad traits of character, of one's motives and desires for being a nurse, of one's ideas regarding the role of a nurse and of the ends of nursing are all important topics for self-reflection.

Nursing as a practice: Its internal goods and the virtues

MacIntyre's conception of a practice is complex. Is nursing a practice in MacIntyre's view? In other words, is nursing a complex and coherent form of socially established cooperative human activity? I could easily assert that nursing is complex; after all, I am a nurse. But how is one to evaluate the meaning of 'complex'? The work of contemporary nurses involves many activities and practices, innumerable moral conflicts and dilemmas arise and contemporary nursing practice abounds with complex moral and clinical decisions. Therefore, at this level it seems reasonable to suppose that nursing is a form of complex human activity. I also suggest that nursing is socially established; it is organized at a social and community level and regulated by Government; further-more, given the current emphasis on multi-professional team working, nursing is also a cooperative endeavour. MacIntyre was uncertain whether medicine was a practice; it would have been interesting and fruitful if he had debated this further. Miller[2] also believes that medicine is problematic because of the difficulty in identifying its internal goods. Although in Miller's view, medicine, since it has a definite social goal – to help, heal and care for ill persons – can be seen as a purposive practice. Especially in the light of Miller's distinction between purposive and self-contained practices, it seems to me that medicine qualifies as a practice; it is an example of cooperative human activity and it is coherent in that everyone aims to work towards set ends. Furthermore, medicine is complex because it necessitates a rich understanding of many different academic disciplines, for example, biomedical and social sciences, ethics, law and health care policy. If medicine is a practice, then perhaps nursing is too. Sellman[3] believes that there is a strong case for claiming that nursing is a practice on MacIntyre's view. Sellman claims that the internal goods of nursing could derive from helping others, which is something novices entering the profession often refer to. For example, a recent study using discourse analysis[4] investigated reasons why people want to be mental health nurses as opposed to, for example, general nurses. Six final year undergraduates constructed their own stories. One example is:

> I've enjoyed it so much better than general when I've been going through my training and I really do feel its my type of person is to sit and talk to patients, and you've got time in psyche.[5]

Furthermore, Sellman claims that other internal goods could be important

> for those who can be identified as good nurses and that these inter-nal rewards become apparent as the student of nursing moves from mere performance of tasks to a position of immersion in the wider role of nursing.[6]

It would have been useful if Sellman had managed to explicitly identify another internal good, because although I have an idea of the sorts of things he has in mind, I am not certain about this. Perhaps he was refer-ring to the sorts of values and positive emotions that develop and find expression in more experienced nurses who find an affinity within nursing. If so, these feelings are hard to put into words. It might be possible to identify the internal goods of nursing by asking nurses in, for example, the three empirical studies[7] in Chapter 2 that examined the role of the nurse. The themes that were identified in these studies were:

- The need for nurses to respond to patients as individuals;
- The need for nurses to demonstrate respect towards patients;
- The need for nurses to make themselves available to patients;
- The need for nurses to voluntarily decide to spend time with patients, ask them questions and listen to their responses;
- The need for nurses to demonstrate certain 'qualities', i.e., moral virtues such as kindness, patience and honesty.

Perhaps some or all of these are candidates for the internal goods of nursing. Of course, the above objectives could also be achieved through, for example, being a doctor or a physiotherapist. Another way to ask the question is to ask 'What counts as doing nursing well?' In the literature in Chapter 2 regarding being a good nurse, the virtues were at the core of these descriptions. I believe that the internal goods of nursing relate to the emotional responses and feelings in a nurse when she acts, thinks and feels in morally virtuous ways; when she recognizes and believes that her nursing care is morally (and clinically) excellent because of the virtues; when through kindness and patience (and perhaps courage) a nurse works hard to alleviate a patient's pain; when through patience, industriousness and kindness a nurse succeeds in helping a patient to sleep; and when through kindness, patience and gentleness a nurse succeeds in healing a patient's pressure sore. As noted earlier, other people admire and praise virtuous people, but nurses ought to feel proud of themselves when they exercise the virtues to help patients fare well during and beyond illness. When the virtues are exercised, these feelings – the internal goods of nursing – are achieved and the practice of nursing is sustained.

MacIntyre claims that individuals cannot decide what acting well means to them; instead acting well is to be conceived in terms of the particular practices. MacIntyre would reject the idea that an individual nurse can and should work out her own conception of acting well and the good. These aims need to be achieved with reference to the practice of nursing and the team of nurses working on the ward. According to MacIntyre, there needs to be a shared conception of the good and agreement on what the ends of nursing should be and what the internal goods of nursing are. How does a nurse know what a virtue is or which traits of character are virtues? I discussed this question in detail in Chapter 8. In tandem with the use of judgement and moral wisdom, a nurse needs to understand how a particular trait of character relates to and promotes the practice of nursing or the specific activity that forms part of the practice of nursing. In MacIntyre's view, the virtues, for example, kindness and justice will sustain the practice of nursing. Exercising the virtues will help nurses to achieve the internal goods of nursing. Self-reflection and reflection on the role of a nurse and the internal goods of nursing will help nurses to identify which traits are virtues. The virtues will help nurses to search or 'go on a quest' for the good life. For example, nurses can ask questions about the nature of being a good nurse, the meaning and nature of good nursing care and how good interpersonal responses can be formed and sustained. Nurses will see that exercising the virtues has a positive impact on the lives of patients and virtuous nurses will achieve the internal goods of nursing and they will see that exercising the virtues is a good way of being a nurse. MacIntyre believes that unless there is a single shared conception of the good life, the virtues will be marginalized. He believes that if the virtues are neglected, if, for example, justice is only understood as a moral principle or obligation, then the virtues will be marginalized and wither away. However, Mason[8] disagrees with MacIntyre. According to Mason, the virtues can still flourish in different practices as long as the individuals within each practice share a conception of the good and cooperate to pursue the good. For example, a team of ten nurses on a medical ward cooperate to exercise the virtues of compassion, courage, kindness, justice and respectfulness. All of the nurses agree that these virtues are crucial to promoting the good, including the survival, recovery and faring well of the patients. While the nurses realize that other virtues will be important given the particular circumstances of each situation, they cooperate to exercise the aforementioned virtues so that they can achieve the internal goods and the practice of nursing is sustained. In Miller's view, a nurse can review the practice of nursing by comparing actions and behaviours with the end it is meant to serve. The standards of excellence relate to the particular ends of nursing. The virtue-based approach to morality with its focus on exercising the virtues helps a nurse to achieve moral excellence. However, I am not saying that acting from obligations means that a nurse *cannot* achieve moral excellence. But in ignoring moral character and neglecting the notion of moral goodness, the obligation-based approach does not facilitate moral excellence; indeed, it seems to me that it facilitates moral competence.

The virtue-based approach to morality as a tradition of enquiry

Regarding the MacIntyrian idea of a tradition of enquiry, each individual nurse is part of a history; one inherits much of who one is from other people. Each person is a bearer of a tradition of enquiry, an intellectual set of ideas – an argument – that situates the practice of nursing. The history of nursing as a profession, the history of nurse education and the histories of everyone entering the nursing profession all operate within a tradition of enquiry. Traditions are dynamic; they change to meet the needs of generations. The virtue-based approach is an example of a tradition of moral enquiry.

Conclusions

I examined MacIntyre's work on the virtues so that I could further situate my account of the virtue-based approach to moral decision-making in nursing practice. I now conceive nursing as a practice on MacIntyre's view although following Miller, I view nursing as a purposive practice because it has clear social goals. The internal goods of nursing are obscure and difficult to articulate. However, fundamentally it concerns nurses wanting to be morally good and wanting to carry out their role to a high moral (and clinical) standard. The positive emotions that one feels, the praise and admiration from others and the memorable sense of achievement that one gains from acting well are, in my view, plausible candidates for the internal goods of nursing. These feelings and responses cannot be achieved by other means. Effectively, the internal goods of nursing are to be found in acting from the virtues and specifically, through the development and sustenance of a virtue-based helping relationship. The virtue-based approach to nursing practice is a tradition of enquiry; the practice of nursing is contextualized and situated within the virtue-based approach to morality. Nurses can identify the virtues in a number of ways, for example, by thinking hard about the conception of a virtue given in Chapter 3, by reflecting on the role of a nurse and by developing a shared conception of the good life. Exercising the virtues of, for example, justice, kindness, patience and courage helps nurses to achieve the internal goods of nursing. Furthermore, exercising the virtues will contribute to the sustenance of the practice of nursing, the achievement of the internal goods and prevent the marginalization of the virtues.

11
Conclusions

Introduction

In this final Chapter, I will summarize the book's argument and reiterate several major problems of the virtue-based approach to morality in contemporary nursing. I will consider some points for further enquiry and research. Finally, I will highlight some of the merits of the virtue-based approach and I will examine the topic of moral education.

The book summarized

Different severities of illness affect people throughout their lifespan; illness forms part of a person's life, i.e., it is a personal phenomena. People can feel several negative emotions created by illness including anxiety, fear, helplessness, powerlessness and vulnerability. Admission to hospital or being cared for at home can intensify these emotions. Notably, illness will often mean that the sufferer is dependent on others for help; one needs help to fare well during and beyond illness. One of the recognized roles of a nurse is to care for patients and promote their independence. In order to achieve this, the development and sustenance of a therapeutic or helping nurse–patient relationship is crucially important. To facilitate this helping relationship, nurses require several qualities including honesty, kindness, patience and trustworthiness. These qualities are particularly important in the light of the current trend towards collaborative and patient-centred care. More accurately, the aforementioned 'qualities' are examples of moral virtues. Therefore, it is necessary to turn to moral philosophy and examine the nature of the virtues. The virtues were at the core of ancient Greek ethics, most notably in Aristotle's[1] ethics. I conceive a moral virtue as a morally excellent character trait, which disposes the possessor to habitually act, think and feel in morally excellent ways. Because moral virtues are moral excellences, people who cultivate the virtues deserve praise and admiration from others. The virtues differ depending on several factors including one's role and cultural background. Nevertheless, exercising the moral virtues is valuable because the possessor and benefactors tend to do well from virtuous activity. Since the Enlightenment, obligation-based moral theories have become popular and they receive widespread attention in the literature. It is clear that moral obligations and the nature and consequences of actions/omissions are morally important features. However, obligation-based moral theories have several well-established flaws. Regarding consequentialism, these include the difficulty in predicting the actual consequences of actions/omissions and they tend to over focus on the notions of the 'Right' and 'right action'. Furthermore, act and rule consequentialism omit to take seriously several other morally important features. For example, they fail to (1) provide a rich account of moral character; (2) provide a rigorous account of the distinctiveness of persons and the significance of relationships in human life and (3) acknowledge the important role played by emotions in the moral life of people. Some of the well known flaws of deontology are : (1) it does not provide adequate action-guidance until its second premise where it actually specifies what a correct moral obligation, rule or principle is; (2) it over-focuses on the notion of 'right action' rather than on the notion of 'moral goodness'; (3) it fails to tell us how to settle conflicts between moral obligations; and (4) as with consequentialism, it fails to account for the significance of relationships in human life. Because of these serious flaws and omissions, I believe that traditional accounts of obligation-based moral theories are incomplete and inadequate.

The question is 'Where should one turn in order to discover a more complete account of the moral life?' My response is to nominate virtue ethics, the moral theory that has the virtues at its core. Virtue ethics aims to (1) provide a detailed account of moral character, (2) resist making an assumption that moral dilemmas are resolvable and (3) provide a satisfactory account of moral education. Supplementary and strong versions of virtue ethics have been developed in general ethics, however, the latter have not been proposed in professional ethics. This deficit is connected to one of the common criticisms levelled against virtue ethics, namely, that it is unable to provide adequate action-guidance or in other words, it is unable to tell people (nurses) what they ought to do in a moral dilemma. But by thinking about the nature and meaning of the virtue and vice terms and by thinking about Hursthouse's v-rules[2] it turns out that virtue ethics does provide adequate action-guidance; or at least it is as adequate as the action-guidance given by consequentialism and deontology. Therefore, a strong (action-guiding) version of virtue ethics is viable and more plausible than the majority of critics acknowledge. Several other problems, however, afflict virtue ethics including the charge of moral relativism, how virtue ethics accounts for 'excessive virtue' and how conflicts between virtues can be resolved. Despite the recognition that nurses ought to cultivate moral virtues and the plausibility of a strong version of virtue ethics in general ethics, obligation-based moral theories remain extremely popular in nursing practice and nurse education. Possible reasons for their popularity include the compatibility between the empirical epistemological paradigm of medicine and the outcome-centred perspective of consequentialism and the compatibility between rule-based deontological ethics and the rules laid down by institutions such as hospitals. In the nursing literature, the topic of moral character is neglected, instead the deontic approach is widespread, for example, the 'four principles'[3] approach. However, there are numerous disadvantages with traditional accounts of obligation-based moral theories in nursing practice. For example, these theories tend to over focus on the nature and consequences of actions/omissions, they make assumptions concerning the resolution of moral dilemmas, typically they ignore the important role played by the emotions in the moral lives of patients and nurses, they fail to settle conflicts between moral obligations and they neglect to acknowledge or they criticize the role of moral wisdom and judgement in the moral lives of nurses. Some evidence suggests that nurses do not utilize obligation-based ethics, for example, principle-based ethics in moral decision-making. Instead, judgement, intuition and instincts are used to make moral judgements. The virtue-based approach to morality advocates the use of judgement and moral wisdom, i.e., moral perception, moral sensitivity and moral imagination. Morally relevant features of situations include the outcomes of actions, intuitions, moral rights, moral virtues, intentions, motives, religious beliefs, past experiences and clinical information. Morally perceptive nurses are able to see the morally relevant features and discern meaning in them. Morally sensitive nurses assimilate this understanding, act upon it and respond to patients' interests and needs in morally good ways. Moral imagination is utilized by nurses to reflect on what it might be like to be a patient in a specific set of circumstances. Such thoughts can help nurses to identify a broad and diverse range of practices, interventions and activities that can help patients. Three features characterize the virtue-based approach to morality: (1) exercising the moral virtues, for example, compassion (2) utilizing judgement and (3) utilizing moral wisdom. The emphasis is on developing and sustaining a virtue-based helping relationship through which nurses help patients to fare well during and after illness. The virtues are not primarily concerned with right action, but with acting morally well, for example, kindly, justly and patiently. The virtue-based approach *does* take into account the nature and consequences of actions/omissions. But many other features lie at the heart of the virtue-based approach to morality in nursing practice. For example, this approach places a greater degree of emphasis on the moral importance of intrapersonal and interpersonal responses, this approach acknowledges and makes pivotal the important role played by emotion (including moral remainder) in the moral lives of patients and nurses and this approach places a firm emphasis on the crucial role played by judgement and moral wisdom in helping nurses to make morally good decisions. In short, the virtue-based approach can be described as context-dependent, relational and particularist for the reasons stated.

There are several important criticisms of the virtue-based approach to morality within nursing. First, it makes assumptions about the nature of virtues and goodness; second, there is ambiguity and disagreement regarding how the virtues are identified; third, there is uncertainty regarding how to account for excessive virtue, for example, being *too* honest with a patient and fourth, there is the difficulty in knowing how to settle conflicts between virtues. However, this approach also has many merits. These include the compatibility of the virtue-based approach with the language of the virtues and vices used by nurses in practice, the adequate action-guidance provided by the v-rules and the content of the virtues, the wider range of morally relevant features that this approach takes into account, its acknowledgement that some moral dilemmas are irresolvable or tragic, the recognition that in so-called resolvable dilemmas virtuous nurses will feel moral remainder and its firm emphasis on moral education. Moreover, the virtue-based approach acknowledges and addresses the need for a particularist approach to morality and moral decision-making in nursing practice; if we are to achieve 'high-'quality nursing, patient-centred and collaborative care, a deontic and universalist approach to morality is unsatisfactory. Instead an adequate nursing ethics should promote and encourage the use of moral judgement and moral wisdom in moral decision-making. While the philosophical foundation for the virtue-based approach to morality in nursing practice is adequate, the work of MacIntyre further develops this foundation. MacIntyre's account of the virtues as set forth in *After Virtue*[4] is examined within three sections: (1) the role and importance of a narrative conception of the self in morality, (2) the meaning and nature of practices, goods and the virtues and (3) the role and importance of a tradition of enquiry in morality. MacIntyre's account of the virtues is relevant to contemporary nursing practice. For example, his account recognizes the importance of allowing patients to tell their narratives, it acknowledges the importance of interpersonal responses and it realizes that questions about personal identify are fundamentally important, for instance, 'Who am I?' and 'How do I relate to my colleague?' MacIntyre's account is particularist and context dependent; two features that aid its compatibility with the virtue-based approach to morality in nursing practice. Nursing is conceived as a purposive practice; it is a complex and coherent form of socially established human activity that provides social goods and demonstrates human excellences. While it is difficult to articulate the internal goods of nursing, I suggest that these goods relate to nurses feeling certain positive emotions. These emotions occur when nurses act, think and feel in morally excellent ways in an attempt to help patients fare well during and after illness. Examples of the internal goods of contemporary nursing practice include the development and sustenance of a virtue-based helping relationship and the pursuit and implementation of virtue-based moral decision-making. The difficult process of identifying the virtues can be facilitated through reflection on several areas, for example, on the conception of the good, on the role of a nurse, one's motives for being a nurse and the ends of nursing. Nurses who exercise the virtues help to sustain the practice of nursing. The virtue-based approach to morality is conceived as a tradition of moral enquiry and the practice of nursing is contextualized and situated within this tradition of enquiry. Exercising the virtues will prevent the marginalization of the virtues.

Criticisms of the virtue-based approach to moral decision-making in nursing practice

In summarizing the book's argument, I have repeated some of the criticisms levelled at the virtue-based approach to moral decision-making in nursing practice that I examined in Chapter 8. To recap, some of the most pressing criticisms are (a) it makes assumptions about the virtues, moral goodness and the meaning of 'virtuous'; (b) the difficulty in identifying the virtues and the charge of moral relativism; (c) how to account for people exercising a virtue such as honesty to an excessive degree; (d) its failure to provide adequate action-guidance; and (e) its failure to settle conflicts between virtues.

While I responded to these criticisms in Chapter 8, I shall now discuss (d) and (e) again.

Inadequate action-guidance

Supplementary virtue ethics is clearly plausible because it combines two different and important approaches, namely, a deontic and an aretaic approach. I believe, however, that supplementary virtue ethics serves as merely an obligation-based moral theory with a slogan attached to the effect of saying 'don't forget to take moral character into account'. It seems to me untrue to suggest that obligation-based ethics provides adequate action-guidance, while the virtue-based approach to morality cannot. I reject the view that people can derive adequate action-guidance from evaluative and inflexible moral obligations, rules and principles. Responses from a recent Delphi questionnaire study support Hursthouse's[5] claim that adequate action-guidance can be obtained from thinking about the meaning of virtue and vice terms. In this study, the language used by nurses on a daily basis included virtue and vice terms such as 'honest', 'fair', 'well', 'good' and 'care'.[6] The use of such terms helps nurses to know how to *be* and also what to *do*. Based on my nursing experience, it is true to say that (at least some) nurses use language such as 'the nurse acted *badly*', 'as a nurse, I need to provide *good* nursing care' and 'it is important to be *fair* when delivering nursing care'. This language is aretaic in meaning. It has been noted how patients associate 'high' and 'good' quality nursing care with the exercise of moral virtues such as kindness and honesty. It is inaccurate to suggest that the language of the virtues and vices utilized in nursing practice is somehow old fashioned or odd; it is actually very commonplace. Furthermore, Hursthouse's v-rules thesis is simple, yet also inspiring. She is correct to suggest that the virtues and vices prescribe adequate action-guidance, for example, 'do what is *just*', 'be *kind* to patients', 'do not be *unfair* to patients' and 'be *respectful* towards patients'. Hursthouse seems to have developed the v-rules thesis as a direct response to the specific objection that virtue ethics fails to provide adequate action-guidance *because* it does not produce any rules; perhaps one could claim that Hursthouse is making an unnecessary concession to obligation-based ethicists who demand action-guidance in the form of moral obligations, rules and principles. However, Hursthouse demonstrates that virtue ethics does indeed produce rules for action. Moreover, the v-rules provide action-guidance that is at par with, if not to say exceeds, the action-guidance prescribed by the single rule of act-consequentialism or the plurality of rules prescribed by the many forms of deontology.

In relation to the charge of inadequate action-guidance, does discussion of the moral virtues ignore the need for nurses to possess good clinical skills? Cultivating and exercising moral virtues will promote the achievement of morally excellent nursing care. However, nursing is often described as a 'practical activity'. Although I believe that this is a myopic view of the work of nurses, it is to an extent an understandable view because the interventions and practices that form, perhaps, the majority of nurses' work needs to be physically practiced and carried out by nurses. How can the moral virtues help achieve clinical competence? I noted in Chapter 8 that virtue-based moral decision-making, especially the use of moral wisdom, can help nurses to think of a diverse range of activities that can help patients and these activities include effective clinical interventions and pharmacological treatments. The nurse's prime motive is to find ways to help patients fare well during and after illness. Thus what might be called 'clinical nursing' is not ignored even if the focus is just on the moral virtues. Of course another response is to refer to Aristotle's distinction between moral and intellectual virtues (as noted in Chapter 3). Aristotle held that practical wisdom (*phronesis*) and theoretical knowledge (*episteme*) were intellectual virtues. Practical wisdom can be understood broadly to mean the practical skills and abilities required to plan and lead a successful human life. In the context of nursing, skills and abilities that help a nurse to organize, plan and deliver care are important to being a 'good' nurse. In tandem with moral virtues, these skills and abilities will help patients to fare well during and after illness. Theoretical knowledge could also be conceived in a similar way. 'Theoretical knowledge' is a phrase that covers a wide range of disciplines required by nurses to be successful in carrying out their roles. Examples of disciplines include anatomy, physiology, law, ethics, psychology, sociology, politics and philosophical skills such as critical and logical thinking. Furthermore, clinical skills such as taking and recording vital signs, applying a bandage and administering medications are, in my view, examples of practical virtues required to be a good, successful nurse. 'Theoretical knowledge' should be understood as an intellectual virtue for two reasons: first, their relevance to whether patients are able to fare well or not is clearly understood and second, the virtues – both moral and intellectual – all aim at human excellence. In short, the virtuous nurse is concerned with developing and maintaining morally *and* clinically excellent care.

Conflicts between virtues

I believe that conflicts between moral virtues are to be expected given the complexity of human lives; an adequate normative ethics should acknowledge and realize that conflicts between deontic concepts such as moral obligations and principles and the aretaic concept of moral virtues will in part arise because of the subjective nature of human lives and the notion of making judgements and the process of moral decision-making; nursing practice is value-laden and abounds with dense and complex moral dilemmas. Nevertheless, the rich action-guidance available from thinking about the meaning and nature of the moral virtues means that nurses will form a good idea of what to do in difficult situations, plus the v-rules will also contribute to providing action-guidance. Nurses will value different virtues. According to the virtue-based approach to morality, nurses will utilize judgement and moral wisdom to ascertain and comprehend the morally relevant features within specific situations. Depending on the nurse's evaluation of the morally relevant features, she might judge that being just is morally preferable to being kind because she values justice as a virtue more than kindness in this particular situation. The virtues are moral excellences, admirable and praiseworthy character traits that help their possessor and others to lead morally good lives. While I accept that prioritizing virtues might be problematic, the point is that the choice is between two or more different moral excellences; either choice is an example of acting virtuously, i.e., the patient will be helped albeit in different ways. I would accept the criticism more if the choice was between acting from a virtue (e.g. kindness) and acting from a vice (e.g. cruelty); clearly, the former trait is morally preferable to the latter.

Areas for further research and enquiry

Identifying the virtues and understanding conflicts between virtues

Empirical nursing research utilizing a range of research methods such as questionnaires, grounded theory and ethnography could aim to examine a series of topics including how virtues are identified and the value of virtues. Moreover, it would be profitable for researchers to investigate the nature of conflicts between virtues and gather information from nurses and patients regarding their views on these complex phenomena. Further, philosophical enquiry on all of these topics is also needed.

Intellectual virtues, judgement and moral wisdom

In this book, I have neglected to sufficiently examine the role of intellectual virtues in nursing practice and their relationship to moral virtues. While it is clear that moral virtues are crucial to the development of a virtue-based, helping nurse–patient relationship, the role of the intellectual virtues requires further scrutiny. Empirical research and philosophical enquiry regarding how nurses utilize practical wisdom and the role of judgement and moral wisdom in the moral lives of nurses and patients would prove invaluable to the development of a rigorous virtue-based approach to morality in contemporary nursing practice.

The virtues and patients with chronic illness

It should be clear that the virtue-based approach to morality in nursing focuses on the development and sustenance of a virtue-based helping relationship between nurse and patient. While nurses can exercise the virtues in any nursing speciality, the development of this kind of relationship is facilitated over a period of time. Some of the examples used in this book centre on patients with chronic illness such as CRA. Patients with chronic illness such as arthritis, diabetes, asthma and manic depression exploit the true nature of the virtues, provide ideal opportunities for the virtuous activity of nurses and facilitate the development of a virtue-based helping relationship. It seems sensible to suppose that the nature of different nursing environments will have an effect on the opportunity and possibility for a virtue-based helping relationship to be formed in the first place. This relationship might not be so achievable in acute settings where patients are admitted and discharged rapidly. Examples of these settings include day-case surgical wards and outpatient clinics. However, it remains important for nurses to cultivate the virtues irrespective of the environment because acting virtuously, for example, kindly, patiently and justly will remain, irrespective of the nursing environment, examples of acting well.

Merits of the virtue-based approach to moral decision-making in nursing practice

I examined the merits of the virtue-based approach to morality in nursing practice in Chapter 8 and I highlighted these again in the 'Summary' section at the beginning of this Chapter. In this section, I shall list some notable merits and then examine two in more detail.

The merits of the virtue-based approach to morality within nursing practice are numerous but include: (a) in their clinical work nurses utilize the language of the virtues and vices, thus a plausible and adequate nursing ethics should acknowledge this; (b) the important role assigned to consequences in the moral life is recognized, but there is also a focus upon the role played by emotion in the moral life of patients and nurses; (c) reasons for action are identified and examined in terms of the virtues and vices, for example, has someone acted well or badly?; (d) the patient's lived experience of illness is expressed in the form of a narrative; (e) patient-centred and collaborative care is facilitated by the aims of the virtue-based approach; (f) moral dilemmas are not assumed to be resolvable; (g) the notion of 'right action' is not emphasized while 'moral remainder' is; and (h) the subject of moral education is held to be of central importance in morality and nursing ethics.

I shall now discuss (f) and (h) in more detail.

The virtue-based approach to morality and Hursthouse on dilemmas and moral remainder

Nurses who cultivate the moral virtues and appreciate the aims of the virtue-based approach to morality in nursing will be aware that moral dilemmas are either (a) resolvable or (b) irresolvable. But in both kinds of moral dilemma, nurses will feel moral remainder – negative emotions such as regret, anguish, guilt, hurt, loss, despair and remorse. Nurses should realize that it is a sign of a virtuous moral character to feel these emotions. It is morally appropriate to feel these emotions because the virtuous nurse is fully aware of the distressing nature of moral dilemmas for both patients and nurses. Nurses and patients will feel moral remainder during and after their involvement in resolvable and irresolvable dilemmas. Irresolvable dilemmas present when two virtuous persons (nurses) do not know what to do. In the end, both virtuous persons do different things; these situations might involve a conflict between virtues. Despite each act being an example of virtuous behaviour – for example, one is just, another kind – each nurse feels moral remainder. This is intensified because each virtuous nurse evaluates his or her behaviour as less than admirable and far from morally good. In Hursthouse's view both nurses' lives will be marred.[7]

Hursthouse on 'morally right decision/right moral decision'

According to Hursthouse, obligation-based moral theories encourage and promote the conflation of two different meanings that can be given to the phrase 'morally right decision/right moral decision'. Assume that in a moral dilemma the options are x (to coerce a patient to have ECT) and y (to respect the patient's wish to refuse ECT). X is the better option because it is believed that ECT will help to alleviate the patient's depression; x is thought more beneficial than y and therefore x is carried out. Other examples of this sort of dilemma (though they might not be seen as such) include whether to sedate a patient against his will, whether to detain someone involuntarily and whether to respect a patient's decision to refuse life-prolonging chemotherapy. These are examples of 'dynamic' ethical issues that have caught the public attention partly through intensive media attention. But as noted in a recent Delphi study[8], other examples of moral dilemmas abound in nursing, for example, should a nurse allow a patient to leave the ward for an hour and should a patient with mental illness be allowed extra pocket money? Returning to the case in point, the decision to go ahead with the ECT is the 'right moral decision' because it is made on the grounds that y was more harmful. But a different use of this phrase refers to a person doing a morally good deed, one that is motivated from the virtues and deserves admiration and praise. In this case, option x, i.e., coercing a patient into having ECT is clearly not a virtuous or admirable act even though it is considered to be the morally right option of the two; coercing a patient to have a treatment against her will is not a morally good deed and does not therefore deserve praise or admiration from others.

Teaching the virtues

It has been noted how virtue ethics views the moral education of the young to be a crucial aspect of the moral life. I shall consider this issue in the context of nursing practice. There appears to be a neglect of the virtues and virtue ethics in the teaching of nursing ethics to pre-registration nurses. This belief was supported by the findings of a small scale Delphi questionnaire study,[9] which found that 4 out of 11 lecturers from selected departments of nursing in the UK taught virtue ethics to pre-registration student nurses. Instead of the virtues, the focus was unsurprisingly on consequentialism and deontology, moral theories that were taught by 10 out of 11 lecturers. If these findings are supported on a wider scale, then many students will not come into contact with the notions of the virtues and virtue ethics and it is possible that obligation-based moral theories are seen as the *only* approach to nursing ethics. In my recent experience of teaching ethics to common foundation programme (CFP) and adult branch pre-registration nursing students, the majority of students had never heard the phrase 'the virtues'. However, further discussion revealed that the students were familiar with traits such as 'patience', 'justice' and 'honesty' and they understood how exercising these traits were crucial to being a 'good' nurse.[10] Typically, students attend lectures, seminars and case studies which serve to provide them with an understanding of the essential issues within the field of nursing ethics. But in the above Delphi study, no specialist lecturers in ethics were employed to teach ethics to students of nursing; this fact might help to explain the lack of focus on the virtues and virtue ethics.

Can the virtues be taught?

In ancient Greece, virtue was understood to be a form of knowledge. Nowadays, it is common to believe that 'knowledge' is something that can be taught. Lutzen and Barbosa da Silva claim that the 'virtues can be learned by anyone'.[11] More recently, Begley[12] has claimed that different educational approaches are required in order to teach virtue and the virtue-centred approach to ethics. In her view, nurse educationalists need to teach more than just theoretical ethics if virtue is to be taught. She claims that nurse educationalists need to facilitate the acquisition of practical wisdom and excellences of character and that virtue, understood by her to mean skills or types of knowledge, can be taught best through a multifaceted humanities approach to nurse education. However, one might argue that the virtues cannot be taught, for example, some people might believe that one is born either 'good or bad' and that is how people remain. Or perhaps, while character change on a major scale might be thought impossible, more 'minor' changes in character such as improving one's self-control might be considered possible. Character change, whether major or minor, is clearly not a simple process, one that can happen overnight; it will take a lot of hard work for someone to change character. I imagine that changing one's character is one of the hardest things a person could ever do. If it is possible to teach the virtues then how might this occur? First, in ethics education, it is common to deliver a series of 'key' lectures followed by smaller group work, for example, seminars, case studies and tutorials. The virtues and the virtue-based approach to morality in nursing practice could all be taught in the same manner; discussion and debate could centre on the nature of virtues, the role of virtues in nursing practice and some common merits and criticisms of the virtue-based approach could be examined. Furthermore, differences between the virtue-based and the obligation-based approaches could be examined and even novice nurses could begin to think seriously about the role of the virtues and vices in nursing practice. Second, the virtues are best demonstrated in the clinical environment, where learners can observe experienced nurses carrying out their roles in a morally (and clinically) excellent manner. However, there is the question of who should judge moral excellence in nurses? This is more problematic than identifying clinically excellent nurses – the latter can be observed and evaluated by using quantitative methods. It is more difficult though not impossible to evaluate a nurse's moral goodness. Despite this obstacle, the notion of positive role models runs deep in contemporary culture and specifically within nurse education.[13] Currently, the notion of 'mentorship' is valued greatly within contemporary nursing practice and education. This is related to a feature of virtue ethics that I mentioned earlier, namely, that in a moral quandary it is often invaluable to ask a wise person for moral guidance. In my nursing experience, it was common for nurses to ask each other for guidance. Indeed, asking colleagues for guidance is usually considered to be a sign of a nurse who is able to work well within a team. Once role models have been identified, the hard work can begin, but although it is a difficult endeavour I concur with Aristotle who believed that cultivating the virtues is possible and that virtuous behaviour resulted from habit.

Conclusions

I have examined several notable criticisms of act-centred obligation-based moral theories and concluded that these theories are incomplete and inadequate moral theories. I therefore find it perplexing that these moral theories remain so popular and widespread in nursing ethics and practice. I have explored different versions of virtue ethics and I characterized a virtue-based helping relationship. I have presented an account of the virtue-based approach to morality, which focuses on several features that traditional accounts of obligation-based moral theories tend to neglect. These features are (1) exercising the virtues, (2) using judgement and (3) using moral wisdom. These features enable morally good decisions to be made; such decisions are contextualized and particular. The cultivation and exercise of moral virtues is of fundamental importance to the end of being a morally good nurse. The practice of nursing can be sustained if nurses exercise the virtues and achieve the internal goods of nursing. If the virtues are seen solely in terms of moral obligation or principles, then I fear that the virtues will become marginalized. Of major importance to the success of the virtue-based approach is the fact that exercising the virtues is recognized by patients; for example, a nurse who acts kindly, a nurse who is patient and a nurse who is courageous will all be singled out, held in great esteem, praised and admired by both patients and other nurses. Naturally, like other moral theories such as consequentialism and deontology it is possible to identify several major criticisms of the virtue-based approach. However, despite these objections, a strong (action-guiding) version of the virtue-based approach to morality is a philosophically adequate and sufficient nursing ethics. As such, it is now time for nurse ethicists, nurse educators and clinical nurses to take the virtue-based approach to morality in nursing practice much more seriously; this rich approach to morality requires further investigation and it demands our attention.

Notes

1—Introduction

1. Henceforth, for brevity, I will refer to 'moral obligation(s)' but typically I am also referring to 'moral rules' and 'moral principles'; I shall make it clear if this is not the case.
2. R. Hursthouse, *On Virtue Ethics* (Oxford: Oxford University Press, 1999).
3. T. L. Beauchamp & J. F. Childress, *Principles of Biomedical Ethics*, 5th edn (New York: Oxford University Press, 2001).
4. A. MacIntyre, *After Virtue: A Study in Moral Theory*, 2nd edn (London: Duckworth, 1985).

2—Illness, Narratives and the Value of the Nurse–Patient Relationship

1. Besides listening to patients' lived experience of illness and viewing the emerging story as a narrative, qualitative researchers focus on devising appropriate methodologies to gather the views of persons with illness. See, for example: P. H. Bulow, 'In dialogue with time: Identity and illness in narratives about chronic fatigue', *Narrative Inquiry* 2003, **13** (1), pp. 71–77; R. F. Zakrzewski & M. A. Hector, 'The lived experiences of alcohol addiction: Men of Alcoholics Anonymous', *Issues in Mental Health Nursing* 2004, **25** (1), pp. 61–77; T. Clouston, 'Narrative method: Talk, listening and representation', *The British Journal of Occupational Therapy* 2003, **66** (4), pp. 136–142.
2. E. D. Pellegrino & D. C. Thomasma, *The Virtues in Medical Practice* (New York: Oxford University Press, 1993), p. 42.
3. Ibid., p. 43.
4. Crudely, a rational act can be defined as an act that promotes one's interests, aims and goals. See, for example: N. Rescher, *Rationality: A Philosophical Inquiry into the Nature and the Rationale of Reason* (Oxford: Oxford University Press, 1988).
5. See, for example: J. L. Johns, 'A concept analysis of trust', *Journal of Advanced Nursing* 1996, **24**, pp. 76–83; C. Snelson, 'Trust as a caring construct with the critically ill: A beginning exploration', in *The Presence of Caring in Nursing* (ed.) D. A. Gaut (New York: National League for Nursing Press, 1992); E. Peter & K. P. Morgan, 'Explorations of a trust approach for nursing ethics', *Nursing Inquiry* 2001, **8**, pp. 3–10.
6. See, for example: A. Baier, 'Trust and antitrust', *Ethics* 1986, **96**, pp. 231–260.
7. A. Baier, 'What do women want in a moral theory?', *Nous* 1985, **19**, pp. 53–65.
8. This section is drawn from: S. K. Aranda & A. F. Street, 'Being authentic and being a chameleon: Nurse–patient interaction revisited', *Nursing Inquiry* 1999, **6**, pp. 75–82, 76–77.

9. R. Dingwell, A. M. Rafferty & C. Webster, *An Introduction to the Social History of Nursing* (London: Routledge, 1988).
10. D. Armstrong, 'The fabrication of the nurse–patient relationship', *Social Science and Medicine* 1983, **17** (8), pp. 457–460.
11. I. Menzies, 'A case study in the functioning of social systems as a defense against anxiety. A report on a study of the nursing service of a general hospital', *Human Relations* 1960, **13** (2), pp. 95–121.
12. Ibid.
13. C. May, 'Research on nurse–patient relationships: Problems of theory, problems of practice', *Journal of Advanced Nursing* 1990, **15**, pp. 307–315.
14. Armstrong, 'The fabrication of the nurse–patient relationship'.
15. See, for example: I. Orlando, *The Dynamic Nurse–Patient Relationship* (New York: Putnam & Sons, 1961); J. Travelbee, *Interpersonal Aspects of Nursing*, (Philadelphia: F. A. Davis, 1966).
16. The literature on holism and holistic nursing care is plentiful, See, for example: S. Woods, 'Holism in nursing', in *Philosophical Issues in Nursing* (ed.) S. D. Edwards (London: Macmillan, 1998), pp. 67–88. The concept of holism developed as a reaction against the medical model of medicine and has become a major issue in both nursing theory and practice. The notion of holistic nursing care carries with it some well-recognized conceptual problems, for example, what is the difference between strong and weak conceptions of holism? Whenever the meaning of a concept is in doubt, it is less likely that a shared meaning can be attained. Further problems can then arise in nursing practice, for example, even if agreement is reached on the meaning of holistic nursing practice and how it can be evaluated, how might we know whether two nurses are each practising holistic nursing care? Nevertheless, at the core of the notion of 'holism' lies a plausible and attractive idea: that patients are not just physical entities. In order to meet a contemporary definition of a 'good' nurse, it is necessary for nurses to care for the 'whole' person including physical, psychological, spiritual and social needs.
17. Pellegrino & Thomasma, *The Virtues in Medical Practice*, p. 42.
18. Ibid., p. 43.
19. See, for example: C. Bulsara, A. Ward & D. Joske, 'Haematological cancer patients: Achieving a sense of empowerment by the use of strategies to control illness', *Journal of Clinical Nursing* 2004, **13** (2), pp. 251–258; S. L. Tsay & L. O. Hung, 'Empowerment of patients with end stage renal disease – A randomized controlled trial', *International Journal of Nursing Studies* 2004, **41** (1), pp. 59–65.
20. See, for example: P. J. Barker, 'The tidal model: The lived-experience in person-centred mental health nursing care', *Nursing Philosophy* 2001, **2**, pp. 213–223; P. J. Barker, M. Leamy & C. Stevenson, 'The philosophy of empowerment', *Mental Health Nursing* 2000, **20** (9), pp. 8–12.
21. Barker, 'The tidal model: The lived-experience in person-centred mental health nursing care', pp. 213–223.
22. See, for example; A. N. Malaviya, 'Outcome measures in rheumatoid arthritis', *Journal of Rheumatology* 2003, **6** (2), pp. 178–183.
23. Department of Health, *The Mental Health Act* (London: DoH, 1983).
24. E. Latvala, S. Janhonen & K. E. Wahlberg, 'Patient initiatives during the assessment and planning of psychiatric nursing in a hospital environment', *Journal of Advanced Nursing* 1999, **29** (1), pp. 64–71.

25. See, for example: M. Hunter, 'Rehabilitation in cancer care: A patient-focused approach', *European Journal of Cancer Care* 1998, **7** (2), pp. 85–87;
26. S. Tilley, 'Notes on narrative knowledge in psychiatric nursing', *Journal of Psychiatric & Mental Health Nursing*, 1995, **2** (4), pp. 217–226.
27. Department of Health, *Working in Partnership* (London: DoH, 1994).
28. F. Nightingale, *Notes on Nursing: What It Is and What It Is Not* (New York: Dover Publications, 1969).
29. D. Lacey, 'Using Orem's model in psychiatric nursing', *Nursing Standard* 1993, **7** (29), pp. 28–30.
30. K. Murphy, A. Cooney, D. Casey, M. Connor, J. O'Connor & B. Dineen, 'The Roper, Logan and Tierney model: Perceptions and operationalization of the model in psychiatric nursing within a health board in Ireland', *Journal of Advanced Nursing* 2000, **31** (6), pp. 1333–1341.
31. Barker, 'The tidal model: The lived-experience in person-centred mental health nursing care', pp. 213–223.
32. H. Peplau, *Interpersonal Relations in Nursing* (New York: Putnam, 1952).
33. M. Musker & M. Byrne, 'Applying empowerment in mental health practice', *Nursing Standard* 1997, **11** (31), pp. 45–47.
34. See, for example: A. Monaghan, 'Communication', in *Potter and Perry's Foundations in Nursing Theory and Practice* (ed.) H. B. M. Heath (London: Mosby, 1995), pp. 275–297; D. Skidmore, 'Communication', in *A Textbook of Psychiatric and Mental Health Nursing* (eds) J. I. Brooking, S. A. H. Ritter & B. L. Thomas (Edinburgh: Churchill Livingstone, 1992), pp. 249–259; S. Speedy, 'The Therapeutic Alliance', in *Advanced Practice in Mental Health Nursing* (eds) M. Clinton & S. Nelson (Oxford: Blackwell Science, 1999), pp. 59–76; H. Wright, 'The Therapeutic Relationship', in *Mental Health Nursing* (eds) H. Wright & M. Giddey (London: Chapman & Hall, 1993), pp. 3–9; O. Ironbar & A. Hooper, *Self Instruction in Mental Health Nursing*, 2nd edn (London: Balliere Tindall, 1989).
35. Ironbar and Hooper, *Self Instruction in Mental Health Nursing*, p. 18.
36. Wright, 'The Therapeutic Relationship', pp. 3–9.
37. Monaghan, 'Communication', pp. 275–297.
38. Skidmore, 'Communication', pp. 249–259.
39. R. J. Gregory, 'Recovery from depression associated with Guillain Barre Syndrome', *Issues in Mental Health Nursing* 2003, **24** (2), pp. 129–135; G. Archibald, 'Patient's experiences of hip fracture', *Journal of Advanced Nursing* 2003, **44** (4), pp. 385–392.
40. See, for example: J. B. Hopkinson, C. E. Hallet & K. A. Luker, 'Caring for dying people in hospital', *Journal of Advanced Nursing* 2003, **44** (5), pp. 525–532; on the notion of 'dignity' and a good death, see: I. Randers & A. C. Mattrasson, 'Autonomy and integrity: Upholding older adult patients' dignity', *Journal of Advanced Nursing* 2004, **45** (1), pp. 63–71.
41. Monaghan, 'Communication', pp. 275–297.
42. A. E. Armstrong, S. Parsons & P. J. Barker, 'Unpublished research findings from a Delphi study investigating moral reasoning in mental health nurses', University of Newcastle upon Tyne, 1999.
43. A. E. Armstrong, S. Parsons & P. J. Barker, 'An inquiry into moral virtues, especially compassion, in psychiatric nursing: Findings from a Delphi study', *Journal of Psychiatric and Mental Health Nursing* 2000, **7**, pp. 297–306.

44. According to holism, all human needs – physical, psychological, emotional, spiritual and sexual – should be taken into account; see: S. Earle, 'Disability, facilitated sex and the role of the nurse', *Journal of Advanced Nursing* 2001, **36** (3), pp. 433–440.
45. See: Nursing and Midwifery Council, *The NMC Code of Professional Conduct: Standards for Conduct, Performance and Ethics* (London: NMC, 2004); Nursing and Midwifery Council, *What Accountability Is* (London: NMC, 2002).
46. Armstrong et al., 'Unpublished research findings from a Delphi study investigating moral reasoning in mental health nurses', 1999.
47. L. Walker, P. J. Barker & P. Pearson, 'The required role of the psychiatric-mental health nurse in primary health care: An augmented Delphi study', *Nursing Inquiry* 2000, **7**, pp. 91–102.
48. H. Peplau, *Interpersonal Relations in Nursing*.
49. A. Altschul, *Patient–Nurse Interaction* (Edinburgh: Churchill Livingstone, 1972).
50. Walker et al., 'The required role of the psychiatric-mental health nurse in primary health care: An augmented Delphi study', p. 96.
51. K. Edwards, 'A preliminary study of users' and nursing students' views of the role of the mental health nurse', *Journal of Advanced Nursing* 1995, **21** (2), pp. 222–229.
52. P. J. Barker, S. Jackson & C. Stevenson, 'The need for psychiatric nursing: Towards a multidimensional theory of caring', *Nursing Inquiry* 1999, **6**, pp. 103–111.
53. B. G. Glaser & A. L. Strauss, *The Discovery of Grounded Theory. Strategies for Qualitative Research* (Chicago: Aldine Press, 1967).
54. Barker et al., 'The need for psychiatric nursing: Towards a multidimensional theory of caring', p. 103.
55. Ibid., p. 105.
56. Ibid., p. 105.
57. M. C. Ramos, 'The nurse–patient relationship: Theme and variation', *Journal of Advanced Nursing* 1992, **17**, pp. 496–506.
58. S. Jackson & C. Stevenson, 'The gift of time from the friendly professional', *Nursing Standard* 1998, **12** (51), pp. 31–33.
59. P. Barker & I. Whitehill, 'The craft of care: Towards collaborative caring in psychiatric nursing', in *The Mental Health Nurse: Views of Practice and Education* (ed.) S. Tilley (Oxford: Blackwell Science, 1997).
60. Barker et al., 'The need for psychiatric nursing: Towards a multidimensional theory of caring', p. 107.
61. J. Strang, *The Emotional Labour of Nursing* (London: Macmillan Press, 1982).
62. Barker et al., 'The need for psychiatric nursing: Towards a multidimensional theory of caring', p. 107.
63. S. Bignold, 'Befriending the family: An exploration of a nurse–client relationship', *Health and Social Care in the Community* 1995, **3**, pp. 173–180.
64. See, for example: K. Kadner, 'Therapeutic intimacy in nursing', *Journal of Advanced Nursing* 1994, **19**, pp. 215–218; P. Marck, 'Therapeutic reciprocity: A caring phenomenon', *Advances in Nursing Science* 1990, **13**, pp. 49–59.
65. F. Arnold, 'Structuring the relationship', in *Interpersonal Relationships. Professional Communication Skills for Nurses* (eds) E. Arnold & U. Boggs, 2nd edn (Philadelphia: W. B. Saunders Company, 1995), pp. 75–85.

66. Aranda & Street, 'Being authentic and being a chameleon: Nurse–patient interaction revisited', pp. 75–82.
67. Barker et al., 'The need for psychiatric nursing: Towards a multidimensional theory of caring', p. 108.
68. L. Bowers, 'Ethnomethodology II: A study of the community psychiatric nurse in the patient's home', *International Journal of Nursing Studies* 1992, **29**, pp. 69–79.
69. V. Ming Ho Lau & A. Mackenzie, 'Attributes of nurses that determine the quality of care for mentally handicapped people in an institution', *Journal of Advanced Nursing* 1996, **24** (6), pp. 1109–1115.
70. Altschul, *Patient–Nurse Interaction*.
71. R. Sanson-Fischer, A. Poole & V. Thompson, 'Behaviour patterns within a general hospital psychiatric unit: An observational study', *Behaviour Research and Therapy* 1979, **17**, pp. 317–332.
72. T. Martin, 'Psychiatric nurses' use of working time', *Nursing Standard* 1992, **6**, pp. 34–36.
73. Jackson & Stevenson, 'The gift of time from the friendly professional', pp. 31–33.
74. K. Hurst & D. Howard, 'Measure for measure', *Nursing Times* 1988, **84** (22), pp. 30–32.
75. D. Whittington & C. McLaughlin, 'Finding time for patients: An exploration of nurses' time allocation in an acute psychiatric setting', *Journal of Psychiatric and Mental Health Nursing* 2000, **7**, pp. 259–268.
76. Ibid., p. 263.
77. A. Pearson, 'Trends in clinical nursing', in *Primary Nursing. Nursing in the Burford and Oxford Nursing Development Units* (ed.) A. Pearson (London: Croon Helm, 1988), pp. 1–122.
78. Armstronget al., 'Unpublished research findings from a Delphi study investigating moral reasoning in mental health nurses', 1999.
79. A. E. Armstrong, S. Parsons & P. J. Barker, 'Unpublished research findings from a Delphi study investigating moral reasoning in mental health nurses', University of Newcastle upon Tyne, 1999.
80. P. Beech & I. J. Norman, 'Patient's perceptions of the quality of psychiatric nursing care: Findings from a small-scale descriptive study', *Journal of Clinical Nursing* 1995, **4** (2), pp. 117–123.
81. Ibid., p. 121.
82. A. MacIntyre, *Dependent Rational Animals – Why Humans Need the Virtues* (London: Duckworth, 1999).

3—The Virtues in General Ethics

1. See, for example: T. Irwin, *Greek Ethics* (Oxford: Oxford University Press, 1999).
2. St. T. Aquinas, *Summa Theologiae*, trans. Fathers of the English Dominican Province (London: Burns and Oates, 1920).
3. T. Hobbes, *Leviathan*, (ed.) C. B. MacPherson (Harmondsworth: Penguin, 1985).
4. D. Hume, *An Enquiry Concerning the Principles of Morals*, 3rd edn (ed.) L. A. Bigge & (rev.) P. H. Nidditch (Oxford: Clarendon Press, 1975).

5. I. Kant, 'The Doctrine of Virtue', in *The Metaphysics of Morals* (ed.) M. Gregor (Cambridge: Cambridge University Press, 1996).
6. This has motivated recent work in moral philosophy that aims to forge links between moral obligations and the virtues.
7. This is drawn from: J. Rachels, *The Elements of Moral Philosophy*, 3rd edn (New York: McGraw-Hill, 1999), pp. 175–176.
8. Aristotle, *The Nicomachean Ethics*, trans. D. Ross, (rev.) J. L. Ackrill and J. O. Urmson (Oxford: Oxford University Press, 1980), Bk 2, 5, 1106a17, p. 36.
9. Aristotle, *The Nicomachean Ethics*, Bk 2, 1, 1103a33, p. 28.
10. Plato, *Meno*, trans. W. K. C. Guthrie in *Protagoras and Meno* (London: Penguin Books, 1956), pp. 101–157.
11. 'Knowledge', in *Oxford Compact English Dictionary* (ed.) D. Thompson (Oxford: Oxford University Press, 1996), p. 549.
12. Aristotle, *The Nicomachean Ethics*, Bk 2, 1, 1103a33, p. 28.
13. See, for example: M. Slote, *From Morality to Virtue* (New York: Oxford University Press, 1992); M. Slote, *Morals with Motives* (Oxford: Oxford University Press, 2001); R. Hursthouse, *On Virtue Ethics* (Oxford: Oxford University Press, 1999); J. Oakley & D. Cocking, *Virtue Ethics and Professional Roles* (Cambridge: Cambridge University Press, 2001).
14. E. Pincoffs, *Quandaries and Virtues: Against Reductivism in Ethics* (Lawrence: University of Kansas Press, 1986), p. 78.
15. J. Rachels, *The Elements of Moral Philosophy*, p. 178.
16. Ibid.
17. F. Nietzsche, *Beyond Good and Evil*, trans. Walter Kaufmann (New York: Vintage Books, 1966), part 5.
18. Rachels, *The Elements of Moral Philosophy*, p. 186.
19. I return to discuss the idea of practices in Chapters 9 and 10 in which I argue for a MacIntyrian practice-based account of the virtues in nursing.
20. M. C. Nussbaum, 'Non-Relative Virtues: An Aristotelian Approach', in *Midwest Studies in Philosophy, vol. XII: Ethical Theory: Character and Virtue* (eds) P. A. French, T. E. Vehling Jr. and H. K. Wettstein (Notre Dame: University of Notre Dame Press, 1988), pp. 32–53, 32.
21. See, for example: R. Hursthouse, *On Virtue Ethics* (Oxford: Oxford University Press, 1999); P. Benn, *Ethics* (London: UCL Press 1998); C. Swanton, 'Virtue Ethics and Satisficing Rationality', in *Virtue Ethics – A Critical Reader* (ed.) D. Statman (Edinburgh: Edinburgh University Press, 1997), pp. 56–81; K. Stohr & C. H. Wellman, 'Recent work on Virtue Ethics', *American Philosophical Quarterly* 2002, **39** (1), pp. 49–71.
22. J. Rachels, *The Elements of Moral Philosophy*, p. 178.
23. NMC, *The NMC Code of Professional Conduct: Standards for Conduct, Performance and Ethics* (London: NMC, 2004).
24. See, for example: M. Slote, *From Morality to Virtue*.
25. I discuss the question of how the virtues can be taught in nursing education in Chapter 11.
26. It is interesting to consider the nature of virtues by thinking about what might happen if one lacked the virtue in question. For example, would Robert fare as well if he lacked kindness? Would people he cared for have benefited in quite the same way? Would his work have been noticed in quite the same way?

27. P. Benn, *Ethics*, p. 178.
28. R. Hursthouse, *On Virtue Ethics*.
29. G. E. M. Anscombe, 'Modern moral philosophy' (eds) R. Crisp & M. Slote, in *Virtue Ethics* (Oxford: Oxford University Press, 1997), pp. 26–44, 43.
30. Hursthouse, *On Virtue Ethics*, p. 42.
31. Benn, *Ethics*, p. 174.
32. In this section I remain consistent and assume that the virtues are *morally* excellent and admirable character traits.

4—A Critique of Obligation-Based Moral Theories in General Ethics

1. The phrase 'act-centred' is often used instead of 'obligation-based', for example, by R. Hursthouse, *On Virtue Ethics* (Oxford: Oxford University Press, 1999). These terms are interchangeable and commonly used as such in the literature. I shall use 'obligation-based' because it makes it clear that the motive for action is obligation (in ethics we are concerned with moral obligations).
2. I take the meaning of 'ethics' and 'moral' to be, for the purpose of this book, synonymous. I am aware that the origin of 'ethics' is Greek, from *ethos* meaning custom, and the origin of 'morals' is Latin, from *moralis* meaning good behaviour. I use moral to achieve consistency because both virtues and obligations are referred to by the word 'moral' (not 'ethical').
3. This is of course too crude a description, but it makes an accurate point. However, there are various conceptions of obligation-based ethics; some focus on moral rules and object to moral obligations, while others rely heavily on certain strict *prima facie* obligations. And as is common with moral theories, some versions are strict, others moderate and yet others expressed in weak forms.
4. Kantianism (or Kantian ethics) is not featured in this chapter as a particular, extreme form of deontology. Although it is clearly based on Kant's ethics, differences do exist. Indeed, the distinction between Kant's ethics, Kants's ethics and Kantian ethics is the object of a large body of literature, see for example, O. O'Neill, 'Kant's Ethics', in *A Companion to Ethics* (ed.) P. Singer (Oxford: Blackwells, 1991), pp. 175–185. Crudely, Kantianism is a moral theory that claims that the morality of an act has nothing at all to do with its consequences; it all comes down to the nature of the act itself. Kantians accept several of Kant's claims regarding human morality. For example, the prime role of 'reason' in the lives of people, the range of perfect and imperfect duties people owe to others and the importance of both hypothetical and categorical imperatives in the moral lives of people.
5. Henceforth, I use only 'consequences' for brevity.
6. R. G. Frey talks about act-utilitarianism and act-consequentialism, but makes it clear that these are interchangeable and represent the same theory, see R. G. Frey, 'Act-utilitarianism', in *Ethical Theory* (ed.) H. LaFollette (Oxford: Blackwell Publishers, 2000), pp. 165–182.
7. Ibid., p. 165.
8. J. Glover, *Causing Death and Saving Lives* (Harmondsworth: Penguin, 1977), p. 3.

9. Frey, 'Act-utilitarianism', p. 165.
10. Ibid.
11. J. Griffin, *Wellbeing* (Oxford: Clarendon Press, 1986).
12. Frey, 'Act-utilitarianism', p. 165.
13. For a discussion of value theory including desire accounts of value and the 'best interests standard' used in health care ethics see: D. DeGrazia, 'Value theory and the best interests standard', *Bioethics* **9** (1), 1995, pp. 50–61.
14. R. M. Hare, *Moral Thinking* (Oxford: Oxford University Press, 1981).
15. J. S. Mill, 'Utilitarianism', in *Classics of Western Philosophy* (ed.) S. M. Cahn (Indianapolis: Hackett Publishing Group, Inc. 1990), pp. 1063–114, 1066–1067.
16. J. Rachels, *The Elements of Moral Philosophy*, 3rd edn (New York: McGraw-Hill, 1999), p. 189.
17. B. Williams, *Ethics and the Limits of Philosophy* (Cambridge, MA: Harvard University Press, 1985); B. Williams, *Making Sense of Humanity* (Cambridge: Cambridge University Press, 1995).
18. R. Hursthouse, *On Virtue Ethics*, p. 44.
19. Ibid.
20. Ibid., p. 45.
21. Ibid.
22. Ibid.
23. Ibid.
24. Ibid., p. 46.
25. Ibid.
26. Ibid.
27. Ibid.
28. Ibid.
29. Ibid.
30. Ibid., p. 47.
31. Ibid.
32. Ibid.
33. Ibid.
34. Ibid., p. 26.
35. Ibid., p. 27.
36. Ibid., p. 31.
37. Ibid., p. 55.
38. Ibid.
39. Ibid.
40. Ibid.
41. M. Stocker, 'The Schizophrenia of Modern Ethical Theories', in *Virtue Ethics* (eds) R. Crisp & M. Slote (Oxford: Oxford University Press, 1997), pp. 66–78.
42. Ibid., p. 74.
43. Ibid.
44. Frey, 'Act-utilitarianism', p. 166.
45. Ibid.
46. J. S. Mill, 'Utilitarianism' (ed.) R. Crisp, in *Utilitarianism* (Oxford: Oxford University Press, 1998).
47. Rachels, *The Elements of Moral Philosophy*, p. 18.

48. Ibid.
49. The charge that act-consequentialism produces conflicts and clashes with at least some of our moral intuitions, though standard since Hare's (1981) *Moral Thinking*, remains unsettled. Thus the question of whether moral intuitions possess probative force (i.e., the ability to prove x or y) in ethics remains disputed. Morality is not definable by empirical facts unlike the human sciences. This is a crude claim that raises complex but crucial epistemological issues and questions that require critical scrutiny. Much depends upon whether one is an advocate of moral realism or not, but even this apparently simple division is not as simple as it might appear.
50. J. Rawls, *A Theory of Justice* (Cambridge, MA: Harvard University Press, 1971).
51. Frey, 'Act-utilitarianism', p. 167.
52. H. Sidgwick, *The Methods of Ethics* (London: Macmillan, 1962).
53. J. J. C. Smart, 'An outline of a system of utilitarian ethics', in *Utilitarianism For and Against* (Cambridge: Cambridge University Press, 1973), pp. 3–67.
54. E. Pincoffs, 'Quandary Ethics', in *Ethical Theory 2 – Theories about How We Should Live* (ed.) J. Rachels (New York: Oxford University Press, 1998), pp. 187–205.
55. Hursthouse, *On Virtue Ethics*, pp. 39–40.
56. Frey, 'Act-consequentialism', p. 168.
57. D. Lyons, *Forms and Limits of Utilitarianism* (Oxford: Oxford University Press, 1965).
58. 'Rule Utilitarianism', in *The Internet Encyclopaedia of Philosophy* (author unknown), www.utm.edu/research/iep/r/ruleutil.htm, last accessed 12/1/02.
59. 'Deontology' derives from the Greek *'deon'* translated as 'duty'.
60. This section is based on: Nancy (Ann) Davis, 'Contemporary deontology', in *A Companion to Ethics* (ed.) P. Singer (Oxford: Blackwell Publishers, 1990), pp. 205–218.
61. Ibid., p. 205.
62. J. Rawls, *A Theory of Justice*, p. 24.
63. Ibid., p. 30.
64. Ibid.
65. C. Fried, *Right and Wrong* (Cambridge, MA: Harvard University Press, 1978), p. 9.
66. Davis, 'Contemporary deontology', p. 206.
67. Ibid., pp. 206–207.
68. Ibid., p. 207.
69. Ibid.
70. I made this point earlier in the section on 'Consequentialism'.
71. Davis, 'Contemporary deontology', p. 207.
72. Ibid.
73. Fried, *Right and Wrong*, pp. 9–10.
74. This is a strand of thought debated by moral particularism and universalism.
75. T. Nagel, *The View from Nowhere* (New York: Oxford University Press, 1986), p. 177.
76. Davis, 'Contemporary deontology', p. 209.
77. Ibid.
78. Fried, *Right and Wrong*, p. 13.

79. Ibid.
80. Davis, 'Contemporary deontology', p. 209.
81. Nagel, *The View from Nowhere*, p. 179.
82. Davis, 'Contemporary deontology', p. 210.
83. Nagel, *The View from Nowhere*, p. 176.
84. A. Donagan, *The Theory of Morality* (Chicago: University of Chicago Press, 1977), p. 66.
85. Hursthouse, *On Virtue Ethics*, p. 53.
86. Davis, 'Contemporary deontology', p. 212.
87. Hursthouse, *On Virtue Ethics*, p. 27.
88. Ibid.
89. W. Frankena, *Ethics* (NJ, USA: Prentice Hall, 1973) cited in R. Hursthouse, *On Virtue Ethics*, p. 27.
90. Hursthouse, *On Virtue Ethics*, p. 31.
91. Ibid.
92. Davis, 'Contemporary deontology', p. 213.
93. Ibid.
94. Donagan, *The Theory of Morality*, p. 183.
95. Davis, 'Contemporary deontology', p. 213.
96. Fried, *Right and Wrong*, p. 10.
97. Davis, 'Contemporary deontology', p. 216.
98. Hursthouse, *On Virtue Ethics*, p. 33.
99. Ibid., p. 62.
100. See, for example: B. Almond, 'Rights', in *A Companion to Ethics* (ed.) P. Singer (Oxford: Blackwells, 1991), pp. 259–269; L. Sumner, *The Moral Foundation of Rights* (Oxford: Clarendon Press, 1987).
101. See, for example: Department of Health, *The Patients Charter* (London: DoH, 1992); Department of Health, *The Patients Charter and You* (London: DoH, 1999); NMC, *The Code of Professional Conduct: Standards for Conduct, Performance and Ethics* (London: NMC, 2004); Department of Health, *The Human Rights Act* (London: DoH, 1998).
102. P. Jones, *Rights* (London: Macmillan, 1994).
103. Hursthouse, *On Virtue Ethics*, pp. 53–54.
104. Ibid., p. 54.
105. O. O'Neill, *Abstraction, Idealization and Ideology in Ethics* (Cambridge: Cambridge University Press, 1987) cited in R. Hursthouse, *On Virtue Ethics*, p. 54.
106. Ibid.
107. S. Scheffler, *Human Morality* (Oxford: Oxford University Press, 1992, p. 43) cited in R. Hursthouse, *On Virtue Ethics*, p. 54.

5—The Origins, Development and Tenets of Virtue Ethics

1. G. E. M. Anscombe, 'Modern Moral Philosophy', in *Virtue Ethics* (eds) R. Crisp & M. Slote (Oxford: Oxford University Press, 1997).
2. J. Rachels, *The Elements of Moral Philosophy*, 3rd edn (New York: McGraw Hill, 1999), p. 177.

3. See, for example: Aristotle, *The Nicomachean Ethics*, trans. D. Ross, revised J. L. Ackrill & J. O. Urmson (Oxford: Oxford University Press, 1980); M. Slote, *From Morality to Virtue* (New York: Oxford University Press, 1992); M. Slote, 'Agent-Based Virtue Ethics', in *Virtue Ethics* (eds) R. Crisp & M. Slote (Oxford: Oxford University Press, 1997); and R. Hursthouse, *On Virtue Ethics* (Oxford: Oxford University Press, 1999).
4. G. Pence, 'Virtue Theory', in *A Companion to Ethics* (ed.) P. Singer (Oxford: Blackwells, 1991), pp. 249–258.
5. Rachels, *The Elements of Moral Philosophy*, pp. 189–193.
6. E. D. Pellegrino & D. C. Thomasma, *The Virtues in Medical Practice* (New York: Oxford University Press, 1993).
7. Pellegrino and Thomasma's version of virtue ethics applied to medicine is best explored and viewed in the light of two previous texts that together develop a substantial philosophy of medicine. See: E. D. Pellegrino & D. C. Thomasma, *A Philosophical Basis of Medical Practice* (New York: Oxford University Press, 1981) and Pellegrino & Thomasma, *For the Patient's Good* (New York: Oxford University Press, 1988).
8. J. K. Brody, 'Virtue ethics, caring and nursing', *Scholarly Inquiry of Nursing Practice*, 1988, **2** (2), pp. 87–96.
9. K. Lutzen & A. Barbosa da Silva, 'The role of virtue ethics in psychiatric nursing', *Nursing Ethics*, 1996, **3** (3), pp. 202–211.
10. A. McKie & J. Swinton, 'Community, culture and character: The place of the virtues in psychiatric nursing practice', *Journal of Psychiatric and Mental Health Nursing*, 2000, **7**, pp. 35–42.
11. A. M. Begley, 'Practising virtue: A challenge to the view that a virtue centred approach to ethics lacks practical content', *Nursing Ethics* 2005, **12**, pp. 622–637.
12. Lutzen & Barbosa da Silva, 'The role of virtue ethics in psychiatric nursing', p. 202.
13. Ibid.
14. Ibid., p. 203.
15. Ibid., p. 210.
16. M. S. Kashka & P. K. Keyser, 'Ethical issues in informed consent and ECT', *Perspectives in Psychiatric Care*, 1995, **31**, pp. 15–21, 18.
17. Pence, 'Virtue Theory', p. 253.
18. Rachels, *The Elements of Moral Philosophy*, p. 189.
19. Aristotle, *The Nicomachean Ethics*, Bk 1, 1, p. 1.
20. Aristotle, *The Nicomachean Ethics*.
21. P. Benn, *Ethics* (London: UCL Press, 1998).
22. Benn, *Ethics*, pp. 161–162.
23. Ibid.
24. See, for example: D. B. Ramussen, 'Human Flourishing and the Appeal to Human Nature', in *Human Flourishing* (eds) E. F. Paul, F. D. Miller Jr. & J. Paul (New York: Cambridge University Press, 1999), pp. 1–43.
25. Aristotle, *Nicomachean Ethics*, Bk 1, 7, p. 14.
26. Ibid., p. 13.
27. When Aristotle uses 'best' to describe a life, I think he refers to the sort of life that displays many moral and intellectual excellences, i.e., many moral and

non-moral virtues. Since for him, virtue is determined by a rational principle, which men with practical wisdom (one of the intellectual virtues) can discern, it makes sense that a life of theoretical contemplation, e.g., the life of a philosopher should serve for him as the best life to lead. However, while it is commonly stated that achieving one's potential is a good and of value irrespective of the goals or standards attained, I believe that Aristotle on this conception would not offer praise to someone who, for example, achieved their highest mark of 42% in a maths paper. Would Aristotle claim that this is excellence of reasoning?

28. Skinner (the behaviourist) used exactly the same kind of definition of 'goodness' in his 'reinforcement theory'; see B. F. Skinner, *Science and Human Behaviour* (New York: Macmillan, 1953).
29. Benn, *Ethics*, p. 180.
30. See P. M. Churchland, *Matter and Consciousness* (Cambridge, MA: The MIT Press, 1990), esp. Chapter 2.
31. Benn, *Ethics*, p. 181.
32. Aristotle, *The Nicomachean Ethics*, Bk II, 6, p. 37.
33. Ibid., p. 38.
34. Ibid., p. 45.
35. Ibid., p. 46.
36. Ibid.
37. Benn, *Ethics*, p. 180.
38. Aristotle, *The Nicomachean Ethics*, Bk II, 5, p. 35.
39. Benn, *Ethics*, p. 167.
40. Ibid.
41. Ibid., p. 163.
42. Ibid.
43. Ibid.
44. This is surely disputable depending upon one's conception of sport, for example, mammals such as the big cats spend much of their day playing with each other.
45. Hursthouse, *On Virtue Ethics*, 1999.
46. See, for example: Hursthouse, *On Virtue Ethics*, 1999.
47. See, for example, his treatment of neo-Aristotelian virtue ethics in A. MacIntyre, *After Virtue – A study in Moral Theory*, 2nd edn (London: Duckworth, 1985).
48. Benn, *Ethics*, p. 167.
49. Ibid.
50. However, one should not think that Kant ignored the role of the virtues in morality. He wrote at length about virtue, believing that agents have a strict, perfect duty to cultivate the virtues in themselves; however, the reason or motive for so doing was not to help agents fare well in life, but rather to abide by the categorical imperative. See: I. Kant, 'The doctrine of virtue', in *The Metaphysics of Morals* (ed.) M. Gregor (Cambridge: Cambridge University Press, 1996). Recently some Kantian moral philosophers and virtue ethicists have refocused on Kant's thoughts on the virtues, and much scholarly activity is now directed in this area.
51. Benn, *Ethics*, p. 173.
52. See, for example: S. Scheffler, *Human Morality* (New York: Oxford University Press, 1992); B. Williams, *Moral Luck* (Cambridge: Cambridge University Press, 1981).

53. Slote, *From Morality to Virtue*, 1992.
54. I refer the reader to: M. Slote, *Morals with Motives* (Oxford: Oxford University Press, 2001) and E. Garrard, 'Slote on Virtue', *Analysis*, 2000, **60** (3), pp. 280–284.
55. `Benn, *Ethics*, p. 170.
56. Ibid.

6—Common Objections to Virtue Ethics

1. R. Hursthouse, *On Virtue Ethics* (Oxford: Oxford University Press, 1999), p. 36.
2. Ibid.
3. Ibid., p. 37.
4. Ibid., p. 38.
5. Ibid.
6. Ibid.
7. Ibid., p. 39.
8. Ibid., p. 3.
9. S. Parsons, P. J. Barker & A. E. Armstrong, 'The teaching of health care ethics to students of nursing in the UK: A pilot study', *Nursing Ethics*, 2001, **8** (1), pp. 45–56.
10. J. Rachels, *The Elements of Moral Philosophy*, 3rd edn (New York: McGraw-Hill, 1999).
11. Ibid., p. 190.
12. See, for example: W. D. Ross, *The Right and the Good* (Oxford: Clarendon Press, 1930).
13. P. Benn, *Ethics* (London: UCL Press, 1998), p. 170.
14. G. E. M. Anscombe, 'Modern Moral Philosophy', in *Virtue Ethics* (eds) R. Crisp & M. Slote (Oxford: Oxford University Press, 1997), pp. 26–44.
15. Rachels, *The Elements of Moral Philosophy*, pp. 189–191.
16. Ibid., p. 191.
17. M. Lessnoff, *Social Contract* (Oxford: Polity Press, 1988); D. Gauthier, *Morals by Agreement* (Oxford: Oxford University Press, 1986).
18. Rachels, *The Elements of Moral Philosophy*, p. 192.
19. Ibid., pp. 189–191.
20. Ibid., p. 191.
21. See, for example, Ross, *The Right and the Good*, 1930.
22. B. Gert, C. M. Culver & K. D. Clouser, *Bioethics: A Return to Fundamentals* (New York: Oxford University Press, 1997).
23. Benn, *Ethics*, p. 170.
24. Ibid., p. 175.
25. Hursthouse, *On Virtue Ethics*, p. 13.
26. P. Geach, *The Virtues* (Cambridge: Cambridge University Press, 1977), pp. 29–30.
27. Rachels, *The Elements of Moral Philosophy*, p. 180.
28. Benn, *Ethics*, p. 177.
29. Ibid.
30. While this might sound promising, does it apply to all the virtues? Does it, for instance, apply to justice? It is difficult to imagine justice *not* operating as a virtue.
31. Benn, *Ethics*, p. 177.

32. Ibid.
33. According to Benn, virtue ethics cannot be free-standing. Instead it requires help from act-centred obligation-based moral theories because impartial moral concerns are more morally important and will override the importance for one of the good life. So, if accepted, this means that (Aristotelian) virtue ethics cannot adequately capture the objectives of these concerns.
34. Rachels, *The Elements of Moral Philosophy*, p. 193.
35. Ibid.
36. Hare's indirect two-level account of utilitarianism counts as a hybrid moral theory. But despite the fact that the second level contains deontological rules, Hare is certainly not viewed as a deontologist. See: R. M. Hare, *Moral Thinking* (Oxford: Oxford University Press, 1981).

7—A Critical Account of Obligation-Based Moral Theories in Nursing Practice

1. See, for example: R. Gillon, *Philosophical Medical Ethics* (John Wiley & Sons: Chichester, 1986); S. D. Edwards, *Nursing Ethics – A Principle-Based Approach* (Basingstoke: Macmillan, 1996); T. L. Beauchamp & J. F. Childress, *Principles of Biomedical Ethics*, 5th edn (New York: Oxford University Press, 2001).
2. A. E. Armstrong, S. Parsons & P. J. Barker, 'An inquiry into moral virtues, especially compassion, in psychiatric nursing: Findings from a Delphi study', *Journal of Psychiatric and Mental Health Nursing* 2000, **7**, pp. 297–306.
3. S. Parsons, P. J. Barker & A. E. Armstrong, 'The teaching of health care ethics to students of nursing in the UK: A pilot study', *Nursing Ethics* 2001, **8** (1), pp. 45–56.
4. See, for example: K. D. Clouser & B. Gert, 'A critique of principlism', *Journal of Medicine and Philosophy* 1990, **15**, pp. 219–236; K. D. Clouser & B. Gert, 'Morality vs. principlism', in *Principles of Health Care Ethics* (ed.) R. Gillon (Chichester: John Wiley & Sons, 1994), pp. 251–266.
5. K. J. Llamas, A. M. Pickhauer & N. B. Pillar, 'Mainstreaming palliative care for cancer patients in the acute hospital setting', *Palliative Medicine* 2001, **15**, pp. 207–212.
6. M. S. Kashka & P. K. Keyser, 'Ethical issues in informed consent and ECT', *Perspectives in Psychiatric Care* 1995, **31**, 15–21.
7. Ibid., p. 17.
8. D. K. Kentsmith, P. A. Miya and S. A. Salladay, 'Decision-making in mental health practice', in *Ethics in Mental Health Practice* (eds) D. K. Kentsmith, P. A. Miya & S. A. Salladay (Florida: Grune & Stratton, 1986).
9. Ibid., p. 6.
10. Ibid., p. 7.
11. J. Hopton, 'Control and restraint in contemporary psychiatric nursing: Some ethical considerations, *Journal of Advanced Nursing* 1995, **22**, 110–115.
12. Ibid., p. 111.
13. Ibid.
14. R. Hursthouse, *On Virtue Ethics* (Oxford: Oxford University Press, 1999), pp. 4–5.
15. P. Chodoff, 'Involuntary hospitalization of the mentally ill as a moral issue', *American Journal of Psychiatry*, 1984, **141**, 384–389.
16. Ibid., p. 384.

17. Ibid.
18. Ibid., p. 386.
19. R. Dworkin, *Taking Rights Seriously* (London: Duckworth: 1978).
20. P. Brown, 'Ethical aspects of drug treatment', in *Psychiatric Ethics* (eds) S. Bloch & P. Chodoff (Oxford: Oxford University Press, 1991), pp. 167–184, 167.
21. I refer the reader to the following five examples of literature: S. Eth & J. Wesley Robb, 'Informed consent: The problem', in *Ethics in Mental Health Practice* (eds) Kentsmith, Miya & Salladay (Florida: Grune & Stratton, 1986), pp. 83–109; M. Ward, 'The consequences of service planning in mental health nursing',in *Ethical Issues in Mental Health* (eds) Barker and Baldwin (Cheltenham: Stanley Thornes, 1997), pp. 127–147; C. Gibson, 'Ethical dilemmas faced by mental health nurses', *Nursing Standard* 1997, **11** (48), pp. 38–40; E. S. Kinion, N. L. Jonke & N. Paradise, 'Descriptive ethics and neuroleptic drug reduction', *Perspectives in Psychiatric Care* 1995, **31** (2), pp. 11–14; P. Tarbuck, 'Ethical standards and human rights', *Nursing Standard* 1992, **7** (6), 27–30.
22. I refer the reader to the following four examples of literature: P. Tarbuck, 'Use and abuse of control and restraint', *Nursing Standard* 1992, **6** (52), pp. 30–32; R. Byrt, 'Moral minefield', *Nursing Times* 1993, **89** (8), pp. 63–66; S. A. Salladay, 'Ethical responsibility in mental health practice', in *Ethics in Mental Health Practice* (eds) Kentsmith, Miya & Salladay (Florida: Grune & Stratton, 1986); S. Loubardias, 'Ethics of electroconvulsive therapy consent', *Rehabilitation Nursing* 1991, **16** (2), pp. 98–100.
23. See for example: A. M. Begley, 'Practising virtue: A challenge to the view that a virtue centred approach to ethics lacks practical content', *Nursing Ethics* 2005, **12**, pp. 622–637; A. M. Begley 'Facilitating the development of moral insight: Teaching ethics and teaching virtue', *Nursing Philosophy* 2006, **7**, pp. 257–265.
24. Typically dilemmas are conceived as morally complex situations, where, irrespective of the decision, some harm is done. See, for example: V. Tschudin, *Ethics in Nursing – The Caring Relationship*, 3rd edn (Oxford: Butterworth Heinmann, 2003), p. 134; B. Marcus, 'Dilemma', in *The Oxford Companion to Philosophy* (ed.) T. Honderich (Oxford: Oxford University Press, 1995), p. 201; T. L. Beauchamp & J. F. Childress, *Principles of Biomedical Ethics*, 4th edn (New York: Oxford University Press, 1994), p. 11.
25. Kentsmith, Miya & Salladay, 'Decision-making in mental health practice', 1986.
26. Loubardias, 'Ethics of electroconvulsive therapy consent', 1991, pp. 98–100, 98.
27. What are interests? Who can possess interests? Can a foetus or only competent adults have interests? Can a 'person' in persistent vegetative state (PVS) have interests? Even if it is accepted that interests are subjective and value-laden entities, it is another thing entirely to evaluate what is 'in the patient's best interests' because several issues are implicated not least conceptions of beneficence and benevolence. It is necessary to critically examine the notion of 'interests' using philosophical not empirical inquiry.
28. H. McAlpine, L. Kristjanson & D. Poroch, 'Development and testing of the ethical reasoning tool (ERT): An instrument to measure the ethical reasoning of nurses', *Journal of Advanced Nursing* 1997, **25**, pp. 1151–1161.
29. See, for example: J. Rest, 'A psychologist looks at the teaching of ethics', *The Hastings Centre Report* 1982, **12**, 29–36.

30. Beauchamp & Childress, *Principles of Biomedical Ethics*, 2001.
31. Edwards, *Nursing Ethics – A Principle-Based Approach*, 1996.
32. Gillon, *Philosophical Medical Ethics*, 1986.
33. Hursthouse, *On Virtue Ethics*, 1999.
34. See, for example: K. D. Clouser & B. Gert, 'A critique of principlism', *Journal of Medicine and Philosophy* 1990, **15**, pp. 219–236; K. D. Clouser & B. Gert, 'Morality vs. principlism', in *Principles of Health Care Ethics* (ed.) R. Gillon (Chichester: John Wiley & Sons, 1994), pp. 251–266.
35. Clouser & Gert, 'Morality vs. principlism', p. 253.
36. Ibid., p. 252.
37. Kantians call moral ideals 'imperfect' duties.
38. Kantians call moral rules 'perfect' duties.
39. See, for example: Gillon, *Philosophical Medical Ethics*, 1986; Beauchamp & Childress, *Principles of Biomedical Ethics*, 1994, pp. 361–365.
40. J. Rachels, 'Punishment and desert', in *Ethics in Practice* (ed.) H. LaFollette (Cambridge, MA: Blackwells, 1997), pp. 470–479; J. G. Murphy, 'Repentance and criminal punishment', in *Ethics in Practice* (ed.) H. LaFollette (Cambridge, MA: Blackwells, 1997), pp. 487–493.
41. T. L. Beauchamp, 'The 'four principles' approach', in *Principles of Health Care Ethics* (ed.) R. Gillon, (Chichester: John Wiley & Sons, 1994), pp. 3–12, 6.
42. Clouser & Gert, 'Morality vs. principlism', p. 253.
43. Taken from: Ibid.
44. The word 'autonomy' derives from the Greek and literally means self-rule.
45. Beauchamp, 'The 'four-principles' approach', p. 3.
46. Support for this claim is found in (a) the breath and depth of literature on the subject (b) the centrality of the notion of autonomy in the teaching of ethics to nurses and other health care professionals and (c) the importance of this notion and associated concepts such as informed consent in research ethics.
47. However this situation was different in the early 19th century when non-maleficence (understood simply as 'do no harm') and beneficence (understood simply as 'to do good') were the physician's primary duties towards his patient. In the early 19th century, the moral weight ascribed to patients' rights of autonomy (though limited compared with today) came beneath the two more fundamental obligations of beneficence and non-maleficence.
48. Department of Health, *The Patient's Charter* (London: DoH, 1992).
49. Department of Health, *The Mental Health Act* (London: DoH, 1983).
50. Beauchamp, 'The 'four-principles' approach', p. 5.
51. Beauchamp & Childress, *Principles of Biomedical Ethics*, p. 121.
52. This problem lies at the heart of the confusion present in attempts to resolve medico-moral problems that appear to turn on the meaning, application and limits of autonomy.
53. J. F. Childress, *Who Should Decide? Paternalism in Health Care* (New York: Oxford University Press, 1982), p. 65.
54. Gillon, *Philosophical Medical Ethics*, p. 61.
55. Kashka & Keyser, 'Ethical issues in informed consent and ECT', p. 15.
56. R. Downie & K. Calman, *Healthy Respect* (Oxford: Oxford University Press, 1994), p. 54.
57. Beauchamp, 'The 'four principles' approach', p. 4.
58. Kashka & Keyser, 'Ethical issues in informed consent and ECT', p. 15.

59. Ibid., p. 17.
60. W. Frankena, *Ethics* (NJ: Prentice Hall, 1973), p. 45.
61. Clouser & Gert, 'Morality vs. principlism', p. 258.
62. A. E. Armstrong, S. Parsons & P. J. Barker, 'Unpublished research findings from a Delphi study investigating moral reasoning in mental health nurses', University of Newcastle upon Tyne, 1999; L. Walker, P. J. Barker & P. Pearson, 'The required role of the psychiatric-mental health nurse in primary health care: An augmented Delphi study', *Nursing Inquiry* 2000, **7**, pp. 91–102.
63. Perhaps surprisingly, when asked about their *moral* motives for action some mental health nurses responded by listing *legal* obligations and statue law, e.g., the Mental Health Act (1983); see: A. E. Armstrong, S. Parsons & P. J. Barker, 'An inquiry into moral virtues, especially compassion, in psychiatric nursing: Findings from a Delphi study', *Journal of Psychiatric and Mental Health Nursing* 2000, **7**, pp. 297–306.
64. NMC, *The Code of Professional Conduct: Standards for Conduct, Performance and Ethics* (London: NMC, 2004).
65. See, for example: M. Healy & J. Iles, 'The establishment and enforcement of codes', *Journal of Business Ethics* 2002, **39** (1), pp. 117–124.

8—Virtue-Based Moral Decision-Making in Nursing Practice

Much of this Chapter is adapted from or heavily influenced by R. Hursthouse, *On Virtue Ethics* (Oxford: Oxford University Press, 1999)

1. A 'good' death in terms of delivering 'high-' quality nursing care might be one that is dignified, i.e., pain free, emotional and spiritual needs met and practical matters organized.
2. Hursthouse, *On Virtue Ethics*, 1999.
3. This claim is supported by several empirical studies including: A. E. Armstrong, S. Parsons & P. J. Barker, 'An inquiry into moral virtues, especially compassion, in psychiatric nurses: Findings from a Delphi study', *Journal of Psychiatric and Mental Health Nursing* 2000, **7**, 297–306. It is also a claim put forward by nurses in teaching and learning sessions in response to the question: 'How do you make moral decisions in nursing?'
4. This is adapted from Hursthouse, *On Virtue Ethics*, 1999.
5. Ibid.
6. T. L. Beauchamp & J. F. Childress, *Principles of Biomedical Ethics*, 5th edn (New York: Oxford University Press, 2001).
7. See, for example: L. Blum, *Friendship, Altruism and Morality* (London: Routledge & Kegan Paul, 1980); P. Nortvedt, 'Sensitive judgment: An inquiry into the foundations of nursing ethics', *Nursing Ethics* 1998, **5** (5), pp. 385–392.
8. K. Lutzen & C. Nordin, 'Structuring moral meaning in psychiatric nursing', *Scandinavian Journal of Caring Sciences* 1993, **7**, pp. 175–180.
9. Ibid., p. 176.
10. Ibid., p. 177.
11. See, for example: P. Nortvedt, 'Sensitive judgment: An inquiry into the foundations of nursing ethics, *Nursing Ethics*, 1998, **5**, pp. 385–392; M. J. Johnstone & S. T. Fry, *Ethics in Nursing Practice: A Guide to Ethical Decision-Making* (Oxford: Blackwells, 2002).

12. Lutzen & Nordin, 'Structuring moral meaning in psychiatric nursing', p. 178.
13. Ibid.
14. Ibid.
15. See, for example: Beauchamp & Childress, *Principles of Biomedical Ethics*, 2001; S. D. Edwards, *Nursing Ethics – A Principle-Based Approach* (Basingstoke: Macmillan, 1996); R. Gillon, *Philosophical Medical Ethics* (Chichester: John Wiley & Sons, 1986).
16. Lutzen & Nordin, 'Structuring moral meaning in psychiatric nursing', p. 179.
17. K. Lutzen & C. Nordin, 'Modifying autonomy – A concept grounded in nurses' experiences of moral decision making in psychiatric practice', *Journal of Medical Ethics* 1994, **20**, pp. 101–107.
18. This claim is supported by: Armstrong, Parsons & Barker, 'An inquiry into moral virtues, especially compassion, in psychiatric nurses: Findings from a Delphi study', 2000.
19. See, for example: L. Cohen, 'Power and change in health care: Challenge for nursing', *Journal of Nurse Education* 1992, **31**, pp. 113–116.
20. If I attempt to put myself into another person's shoes and imagine what it might be like from their perspective, one of the problems is that I take my value and belief system with me. Therefore, I cannot see things from the other person's perspective because I am unaware – have no knowledge of – their values and beliefs. See: S. Z. Jaeger, 'Teaching health care ethics: The importance of moral sensitivity for moral reasoning', *Nursing Philosophy* 2001, **2**, pp. 131–143.
21. By this I simply mean that there are pragmatic reasons that can prevent nurses from asking these sorts of questions and gathering such information. For example, too many nursing activities, too few suitably skilled nurses and insufficient time to deliver the planned nursing care means that nurses do not have a lot of time to spend with patients in order to ask these sorts of questions. Furthermore, the range of interests and needs that patients have is broad; these notions are not simple and require time to identify and accrue knowledge of.
22. J. Oakley, *Morality and the Emotions* (London: Routledge, 1992).
23. On the complex multidimensional notions of empathy and sympathy, see: T. Yegdich, 'On the phenomenology of empathy in nursing: Empathy or sympathy?', *Journal of Advanced Nursing* 1999, **30** (1), pp. 83–93; L. Baillie, 'A phenomenological study of the nature of empathy', *Journal of Advanced Nursing* 1996, **24**, pp. 1300–1308.
24. P. A. Scott, 'Emotion, moral perception and nursing practice', *Nursing Philosophy* 2000, **1**, pp. 123–133.
25. Ibid., pp. 126–127.
26. I. Murdoch, *Sovereignty of Good* (London: Routledge & Kegan Paul, 1970).
27. E. S. Kinion, N. L. Jonke and N. Paradise, 'Descriptive ethics and neuroleptic drug reduction', *Perspectives in Psychiatric Care* 1995, **31** (2) pp. 11–14, 81.
28. L. Blum, 'Compassion', in *Explaining Emotions* (ed.) A. O. Rorty (Los Angeles: University of California Press, 1980), pp. 507–517, 513.
29. Armstrong, Parsons & Barker, 'An inquiry into moral virtues, especially compassion, in psychiatric nurses: Findings from a Delphi study', 2000.
30. Benevolence is often called kindness and Hursthouse calls it by its perhaps more old-fashioned name, charity. Kindness is clearly part of the compassionate nurses' motives. Lutzen and Nordin claim that benevolence could be seen as a moral virtue (I believe it is). In a grounded theory study, benevolence,

the wish to do good, 'appeared as the nurses' genuine intentions verbally expressed, to do that which is judged to be 'good' for the 'other''. See: K. Lutzen and C. Nordin, 'Benevolence, a central moral concept derived from a grounded theory study of nursing decision making in psychiatric settings', *Journal of Advanced Nursing* 1993, **18**, pp. 1106–1111, 1107.

31. E. D. Pellegrino & D. C. Thomasma, *The Virtues in Medical Practice* (New York: Oxford University Press, 1993), p. 80.
32. Armstrong, Parsons & Barker, 'An inquiry into moral virtues, especially compassion, in psychiatric nurses: Findings from a Delphi study', pp. 297–306.
33. K. Lutzen & A. Barbosa da Silva, 'The role of virtue ethics in psychiatric nursing, *Nursing Ethics* 1996, **3** (3), pp. 202–211, 203.
34. Ibid., p. 203.
35. M. Nussbaum, 'Compassion: The basic social emotion', *Social Philosophy and Policy Foundation*, 1996, **13**, pp. 27–58, 37.
36. H. J. Nouwen, D. P. McNeill & D. A. Morrison, *Compassion: A Reflection on the Christian Life* (London: Darton, Longman and Todd, 1982), p. 4.
37. In nursing, this view is shared among others: A. G. Tuckett, 'An ethic of the fitting: A conceptual framework for nursing practice', *Nursing Inquiry* 1998, **5**, pp. 220–227, 221.
38. This is described by Eisenberg and Miller as when an agent deliberately and intentionally helps and supports another agent without expecting any reward or punishment; in other words, the agent puts the interests of the other ahead of his own for virtuous reasons. See: N. Eisenberg and P. Miller, 'Empathy, sympathy and altruism: Empirical and conceptual', in *Empathy and its Development* (eds) N. Eisenberg and J. Strayer (Cambridge: Cambridge University Press, 1987), pp. 292–316, 87.
39. E. von Dietze & A. Orb, 'Compassionate care: A moral dimension of nursing', *Nursing Inquiry* 2000, **7**, pp. 166–174, 174.
40. This is discussed in: V. Tschudin, *Ethics in Nursing – The Caring Relationship*, 3rd edn (Oxford: Butterworth Heinemann, 2003), pp. 1–17.
41. Armstrong, Parsons & Barker, 'An inquiry into moral virtues, especially compassion, in psychiatric nurses: Findings from a Delphi study', pp. 297–306.
42. For the view that caring is a central virtue in nursing see: J. K. Brody, 'Virtue ethics, caring, and nursing', *Scholarly Inquiry for Nursing Practice* 1988, **2** (2), 87–96.
43. See, for example: H. Breen, 'The Psychiatric nurse – Patient advocate?' *Canadian Journal of Psychiatric Nursing* 1992, **31** (4), pp. 9–11; G. W. Martin, 'Ritual action and its effect on the role of the nurse as advocate', *Journal of Advanced Nursing* 1998, **27** (1), pp. 189–194; M. Mallick, 'Advocacy in nursing – A review of the literature', *Journal of Advanced Nursing* 1997, **25** (1), pp. 130–138.
44. Penn thinks that patient advocacy is particularly relevant when caring for patients with palliative care needs, see: K. Penn, Patient advocacy in palliative care, *British Journal of Nursing* 1994, **3**, 1, pp. 40–42.
45. P. T. Geach, *The Virtues* (Cambridge: Cambridge University Press, 1977), pp. 150–170.
46. Reasons for being an advocate include that it is seen as a traditional role of a nurse usually because it is argued that nurses know patients better than other health care professionals and nurses have sufficient knowledge to promote the patient's interests. Reasons against include the idea that being an

advocate can be a risky business and that nurses lack sufficient control and power to be effective advocates. See: J. Hewitt, 'A critical review of the arguments debating the role of the nurse advocate', *Journal of Advanced Nursing* 2002, **37** (5), pp. 439–445.

47. P. A. Cooksley, 'Caring for the Older Person with a Disorder of the Nervous System', in *Watson's Medical and Surgical Nursing and Related Physiology*, 4th edn (eds) J. Royal & M. Walsh (London: Balliere Tindall, 1992), pp. 681–762, 751–753.

48. NMC, *The Code of Professional Conduct: Standards for Conduct, Performance and Ethics* (London: NMC, 2004).

49. No author credited – 'Sinemet', in *Monthly Index of Medical Specialities* (ed.) C. Duncan (London: Haymarket Publishing Services, 2003), p. 112.

50. Downing asserts that the assessment of pain is complex. It needs to be carried out over a period of time to build up a realistic and accurate picture of the pain, its effects on the patient and the efficiency of pain management strategies. The emphasis is therefore upon a nurse who needs to be motivated to ask relevant questions, spend time with the patient, return to the patient again and again and repeat the questions, review the patient's lived experience of the pain, spend time documenting this information in the nursing records and liase with other members of the health care team. The major objective is to work together to alleviate the pain, facilitate coping strategies and promote the independence of the patient. See: J. Downing, 'Palliative care pain', *Nursing Times* 1997, **93**, 34, pp. 57–60.

51. This is recognized as a common side effect of morphine, see No author credited – 'Morphine', in *Monthly Index of Medical Specialities* (ed.) C. Duncan (London: Haymarket Publishing Services, 2003), p. 121. <Not listed in the Reference list.>

52. S. Ahmedzai & D. Brooks, 'Transdermal fentanyl versus slow release oral morphine in cancer pain: Preference, efficacy, and quality of life', *Journal of Pain & Symptom Management*, 1997, **13**, 5, pp. 254–261.

53. Armstrong, Parsons & Barker, 'An inquiry into moral virtues, especially compassion, in psychiatric nursing: Findings from a Delphi study', 2000.

54. Hursthouse, *On Virtue Ethics*, 1999.

55. Ibid.

56. See, for example: A. Kenny, *Action, Emotion and Will* (London: Routledge, 1963); N. Rescher, *Rationality: A Philosophical Inquiry into the Nature and the Rationale of Reason* (Oxford: Oxford University Press, 1988).

57. R. Hursthouse, 'Virtue theory and abortion', in *Virtue Ethics* (eds) R Crisp & M. Slote (Oxford: Oxford University Press, 1997), pp. 217–238.

58. Ibid., p. 227.

59. Aristotle, *The Nicomachean Ethics*, trans. D. Ross, revised J. L. Ackrill and J. O. Urmson (Oxford: Oxford University Press, 1980).

60. M. Slote, *From Morality to Virtue* (New York: Oxford University Press, 1992); M. Slote, 'Agent-Based Virtue Ethics', in *Virtue Ethics* (eds) R. Crisp & M. Slote (Oxford: Oxford University Press, 1997); M. Slote, *Morals with Motives* (Oxford: Oxford University Press, 2001).

61. Hursthouse, *On Virtue Ethics*, 1999.

62. S. Parsons, P. J. Barker & A. E. Armstrong, 'The teaching of health care ethics to students of nursing in the UK: A pilot study', *Nursing Ethics* 2001, **8** (1), pp. 45–56.

63. Hursthouse, *On Virtue Ethics*, 1999.
64. P. Benn, *Ethics* (London: UCL, 1998).
65. R. Norman, 'Aristotle: The rationality of the emotions', in *The Moral Philosophers* (Oxford: Clarendon Press, 1983), pp. 37–55.
66. This example can be seen as an illustration of 'benevolent deception', i.e., the withholding of a piece of information for morally good – benevolent – motives. Since benevolence is a virtue, there will be times when this sort of practice is an example of acting well. Clearly from the virtue-based perspective, there are differences between blatant lying, deception and withholding information. If a nurse lies to a patient without morally good (virtuous) reasons and without the patient asking questions then this will be an example of acting badly. As noted, this is not the same as withholding information. Deceiving a patient sometimes includes an element of withholding information, for example, when the relatives of a patient state that under no circumstances should the patient be told about his diagnosis because they believe that he just could not cope with the news. This might then set in motion a series of deceitful actions, for example, nurses who begin to avoid the patient's questions. These sorts of situations are on a practical and moral level undesirable. Morally speaking, the vice of dishonesty is being exercised; therefore at least some of these situations are examples of acting badly. The relative's motives appear morally good, but no assumptions should be made regarding the sincerity of such motives.
67. See, for example: Benn, *Ethics*, 1998; J. Rachels, *The Elements of Moral Philosophy*, 3rd edn (New York: McGraw Hill, 1999); R. B. Louden, 'On Some Vices of Virtue Ethics', in *Virtue Ethics* (eds) R. Crisp & M. Slote (Oxford: Oxford University Press, 1997), pp. 201–216; P. Pettit, 'The consequentialist perspective', in *Three Methods of Ethics* (Oxford: Blackwells, 1997), pp. 92–174.
68. This is Hursthouse's interpretation in *On Virtue Ethics*, 1999.

9—MacIntyre's Account of the Virtues

This section draws information from five main sources: (1) A. MacIntyre, *After Virtue – A study in moral theory*, 2nd edn (London: Duckworth, 1985); (2) J. Horton & S. Mendus, 'Alasdair MacIntyre: *After Virtue* and after", in *After MacIntyre – Critical Perspectives on the Work of Alasdair MacIntyre* (eds) Horton & Mendus (Cambridge: Polity Press, 1994); (3) D. Miller, 'Virtues, practices and justice', in *After MacIntyre*, pp. 245–264; (4) A. MacIntyre, 'A partial response to my critics', in *After MacIntyre*, pp. 283–304; and (5) A. Mason, 'MacIntyre on modernity and how it has marginalized the virtues', in *How Should One Live?* (ed.) R. Crisp (Oxford: Oxford University Press, 1996), pp. 191–209.

10—MacIntyre's Account of the Virtues and the Virtue-Based Approach to Moral Decision-Making in Nursing Practice

1. J. Horton & S. Mendus, 'Alasdair MacIntyre: *After Virtue* and after', in *After MacIntyre – Critical Perspectives on the Work of Alasdair MacIntyre* (eds) Horton & Mendus (Cambridge: Polity Press, 1994) pp. 1–15.

2. D. Miller, 'Virtues, practices and justice', in *After MacIntyre – Critical Perspectives on the Work of Alasdair MacIntyre* (Oxford: Blackwell Publishers, 1994), pp. 245–264.
3. D. Sellman, 'Alasdair MacIntyre and the professional practice of nursing', *Nursing Philosophy* 2000, **1**, pp. 26–33.
4. J. Moir & C. Abraham, 'Why I want to be a psychiatric nurse: Constructing an identity through contrasts with general nursing', *Journal of Advanced Nursing* 1996, **23** (2), pp. 295–298.
5. Ibid., p. 298.
6. Sellman, 'Alasdair MacIntyre and the professional practice of nursing', p. 28.
7. These were: A. E. Armstrong, S. Parsons & P. J. Barker, 'An inquiry into moral virtues, especially compassion, in psychiatric nursing: Findings from a Delphi study', *Journal of Psychiatric and Mental Health Nursing* **7**, 2000, pp. 297–306; L. Walker, P. J. Barker & P. Pearson, 'The required role of the psychiatric-mental health nurse in primary health care: An augmented Delphi study', *Nursing Inquiry* **7**, 2000, pp. 91–102; K. Edwards, 'A preliminary study of users' and nursing students' views of the role of the mental health nurse', *Journal of Advanced Nursing* **21** (2), 1995, pp. 222–229.
8. A. Mason, 'MacIntyre on modernity and how it has marginalized the virtues', in *How Should One Live?* (ed.) R. Crisp (Oxford: Oxford University Press, 1996), pp. 191–209.

11—Conclusions

1. Aristotle, *The Nicomachean Ethics*, trans. D. Ross, revised J. L. Ackrill and J. O. Urmson (Oxford: Oxford University Press, 1980).
2. R. Hursthouse, *On Virtue Ethics* (Oxford: Oxford University Press, 1999).
3. T. L. Beauchamp & J. F. Childress, *Principles of Biomedical Ethics* 5th (ed.) (New York: Oxford University Press, 2001).
4. A. MacIntyre, *After Virtue – A Study in Moral Theory*, 2nd (ed.) (London: Duckworth, 1985).
5. Hursthouse, *On Virtue Ethics*, 1999.
6. A. E. Armstrong, S. Parsons and P. J. Barker, 'An inquiry into moral virtues, especially compassion, in psychiatric nurses: Findings from a Delphi study', *Journal of Psychiatric and Mental Health Nursing*, 2000, **7**, pp. 297–306, p. 300.
7. Hursthouse mentions a third possibility, which she calls 'tragic dilemmas'. These are irresolvable dilemmas, wherein something really horrible happens, for instance, a person dies and, typically, one or more persons involved emerge 'marred'.
8. See: A. E. Armstrong, S. Parsons & P. J. Barker, Unpublished research findings from a Delphi study investigating moral reasoning in mental health nurses, University of Newcastle upon Tyne, 1999.
9. S. Parsons, P. J. Barker and A. E. Armstrong, 'The teaching of health care ethics to students of nursing in the UK: A pilot study', *Nursing Ethics*, 2001, **8** (1), pp.45–56, pp. 49–50.
10. Unpublished teaching observation. From 120 first year common foundation programme (CFP) students, 75% believed that these traits, which they volunteered to me in a lecture, were very important to being a good nurse.

Although not well versed in the technical language of ethics and virtue ethics in particular, these students understood the value and importance of these traits to the work of nurses and to the aim of delivering morally good patient care.

11. K. Lutzen and A. Barbosa da Silva, 'The role of virtue ethics in psychiatric nursing', *Nursing Ethics*, 1996, **3** (3), pp. 202–211, p. 209.
12. A. M. Begley, 'Facilitating the development of moral insight: Teaching ethics and teaching virtue', *Nursing Philosophy*, 2006, **7**, pp. 257–265.
13. See: Lutzen and Barbosa da Silva, 'The role of virtue ethics in psychiatric nursing', 1996.

Bibliography

Ahmedzai, S. & Brooks, D. 'Transdermal fentanyl versus slow release oral morphine in cancer pain: Preference, efficacy, and quality of life', *Journal of Pain & Symptom Management*, 1997, **13**, 5, pp. 254–261.

Almond, B. 'Rights', in *A Companion to Ethics* (ed.) P. Singer (Oxford: Blackwells, 1991), pp. 259–269.

Altschul, A. *Patient-Nurse Interaction* (Edinburgh: Churchill Livingstone, 1972).

Anscombe, G. E. M. 'Modern moral philosophy', in *Virtue Ethics* (eds) R. Crisp & M. Slote (Oxford: Oxford University Press, 1997).

Aquinas, St. T. *Summa Theologiae*, trans. Fathers of the English Dominican Province (London: Burns and Oates, 1920).

Aranda, S. K. & Street, A. F. 'Being authentic and being a chameleon: Nurse-patient interaction revisited', *Nursing Inquiry*, 1999, **6**, pp. 75–82.

Archibald, G. 'Patient's experiences of hip fracture', *Journal of Advanced Nursing* 2003, **44** (4), pp. 385–392.

Aristotle, *The Nicomachean Ethics*, trans. D. Ross, revised J. L. Ackrill and J. O. Urmson (Oxford: Oxford University Press, 1980).

Armstrong, A. E. Parsons, S. & Barker, P. J. 'Unpublished research findings from a Delphi study investigating moral reasoning in mental health nurses', University of Newcastle upon Tyne, 1999.

Armstrong, A. E., Parsons, S. & Barker, P. J. 'An inquiry into moral virtues, especially compassion, in psychiatric nursing: Findings from a Delphi study', *Journal of Psychiatric and Mental Health Nursing* 2000, **7**, pp. 297–306.

Armstrong, D. 'The fabrication of the nurse–patient relationship', *Social Science and Medicine*, 1983, **17** (8), pp. 457–460.

Arnold, F. 'Structuring the relationship', in *Interpersonal Relationships. Professional Communication Skills for Nurses*, 2nd edn (eds) E. Arnold & U. Boggs (Philadelphia: W. B. Saunders Company, 1995), pp. 75–85.

Baier, A. 'What do women want in a moral theory?', *Nous*, 1985, **19**, pp. 53–65.

Baier, A. 'Trust and antitrust', *Ethics*, 1986, **96**, pp. 231–260.

Baillie, L. 'A phenomenological study of the nature of empathy', *Journal of Advanced Nursing*, 1996, **24**, pp. 1300–1308.

Barker, P. J. Leamy, M. & Stevenson, C. 'The philosophy of empowerment', *Mental Health Nursing*, 2000, **20** (9), pp. 8–12.

Barker, P. J. & Whitehill, I. 'The craft of care: Towards collaborative caring in psychiatric nursing', in *The Mental Health Nurse: Views of Practice and Education* (ed.) S. Tilley (Oxford: Blackwell Science, 1997).

Barker, P. J. Jackson, S. & Stevenson, C. 'The need for psychiatric nursing: Towards a multidimensional theory of caring', *Nursing Inquiry*, 1999, **6**, pp. 103–111.

Barker, P. J. 'The tidal model: The lived-experience in person-centred mental health nursing care', *Nursing Philosophy*, 2001, **2**, pp. 213–223.

Beauchamp, T. L. 'The 'four principles' approach', in *Principles of Health Care Ethics* (ed.) R. Gillon (Chichester: John Wiley & Sons, 1994).

Beauchamp, T. L. & Childress, J. F. *Principles of Biomedical Ethics*, 4th edn (New York: Oxford University Press, 1994).

Beauchamp, T. L. & Childress, J. F. *Principles of Biomedical Ethics*, 5th edn (New York: Oxford University Press, 2001).

Beech, P. & Norman, I. J. 'Patient's perceptions of the quality of psychiatric nursing care: Findings from a small-scale descriptive study', *Journal of Clinical Nursing*, 1995, **4** (2), pp. 117–123.

Begley, A. M. 'Practising virtue: A challenge to the view that a virtue centred approach to ethics lacks practical content', *Nursing Ethics*, 2005, **12**, pp. 622–637.

Begley, A. M. 'Facilitating the development of moral insight: Teaching ethics and teaching virtue', *Nursing Philosophy* 2006, **7**, pp. 257–265.

Benn, P. *Ethics* (London: UCL Press Ltd. 1998).

Bignold, S. 'Befriending the family: An exploration of a nurse–client relationship', *Health and Social Care in the Community*, 1995, **3**, pp. 173–180.

Blum, L. 'Compassion', in *Explaining Emotions* (ed.) A. O. Rorty (Berkley: University of California Press, 1980), pp. 507–518.

Blum, L. *Friendship, Altruism and Morality* (London: Routledge & Kegan Paul, 1980).

Bowers, L. 'Ethnomethodology II: A study of the community psychiatric nurse in the patient's home', *International Journal of Nursing Studies*, 1992, **29**, pp. 69–79.

Breen, H. 'The Psychiatric nurse – Patient advocate?', *Canadian Journal of Psychiatric Nursing* 1992, **31** (4), pp. 9–11.

Brody, J. K. 'Virtue ethics, caring, and nursing', *Scholarly Inquiry for Nursing Practice*, 1988, **2** (2), pp. 87–96.

Brown, P. 'Ethical aspects of drug treatment', in *Psychiatric Ethics* (eds) S Bloch & P. Chodoff (Oxford: Oxford University Press, 1991), pp. 167–184.

Bulow, P. H. 'In dialogue with time: Identity and illness in narratives about chronic fatigue', *Narrative Inquiry*, 2003, **13** (1), pp. 71–77.

Bulsar a, C. Ward, A. & Joske, D. 'Haematological cancer patients: Achieving a sense of empowerment by the use of strategies to control illness', *Journal of Clinical Nursing*, 2004, **13** (2), pp. 251–258.

Byrt, R. 'Moral minefield', *Nursing Times*, 1993, **89** (8), pp. 63–66.

Childress, J. F. *Who Should Decide? Paternalism in Health Care* (New York: Oxford University Press, 1982).

Chodoff, P. 'Involuntary hospitalization of the mentally ill as a moral issue', *American Journal of Psychiatry*, 1984, **141**, pp. 384–389.

Churchland, P. M. *Matter and Consciousness* (Cambridge, MA: The MIT Press, 1990).

Clouser, K. D. & Gert, B. 'A critique of principlism', *Journal of Medicine and Philosophy*, 1990, **15**, pp. 219–236.

Clouser, K. D. & Gert, B. 'Morality vs. principlism', in *Principles of Health Care Ethics* (ed.) R. Gillon (Chichester: John Wiley & Sons, 1994).

Clouston, T. 'Narrative method: Talk, listening and representation', *The British Journal of Occupational Therapy*, 2003, **66** (4), pp. 136–142.

Cohen, L. 'Power and change in health care: Challenge for nursing', *Journal of Nurse Education*, 1992, **31**, pp. 113–116.

Cooksley, P. A. 'Caring for the older person with a disorder of the nervous System', in *Watson's Medical and Surgical Nursing and Related Physiology*, 4th edn (eds) J. Royal & M. Walsh (London: Balliere Tindall, 1992), pp. 681–762.

Davis, N. A. 'Contemporary deontology', in *A Companion to Ethics* (ed.) P. Singer (Oxford: Blackwell Publishers, 1990), pp. 205–218.

Davis, R. C. *The Principlism Debate: A Critical Overview*, www.chass.utoronto. ca:8080/~davis/pd.htm, last accessed 16/8/1998, pp. 1–12.

DeGrazia, D. 'Value theory and the best interests standard', *Bioethics* 1995, **9** (1), pp. 50–61.

Department of Health, *The Mental Health Act* (London: DoH, 1983).

Department of Health, *The Patients Charter* (London: DoH, 1992).

Department of Health, *Working in Partnership* (London: DoH, 1994).

Department of Health, *The Human Rights Act* (London: DoH, 1998).

Department of Health, *The Patients Charter and You* (London: DoH, 1999).

Dingwell, R. Rafferty, A. M. & Webster, C. *An Introduction to the Social History of Nursing* (London: Routledge, 1988).

Donagan, A. *The Theory of Morality* (Chicago: University of Chicago Press, 1977).

Downie, R. & Calman, K. *Healthy Respect – Ethics in Health Care*, 2nd edn (Oxford: Oxford University Press, 1994).

Downing, J. 'Palliative care pain', *Nursing Times*, 1997, **93** (34), pp. 57–60.

Duncan, C. (ed.) 'Sinemet', in *Monthly Index of Medical Specialities* (London: Haymarket Publishing Services, 2003), p. 112.

Dworkin, R. *Taking Rights Seriously* (London: Duckworth: 1978).

Earle, S. 'Disability, facilitated sex and the role of the nurse', *Journal of Advanced Nursing*, 2001, **36** (3), pp. 433–440.

Edwards, K. 'A preliminary study of users' and nursing students' views of the role of the mental health nurse', *Journal of Advanced Nursing*, 1995, **21** (2), pp. 222–229.

Edwards, S. D. *Nursing Ethics – A Principle-Based Approach* (Basingstoke: Macmillan, 1996).

Eisenberg, N. & Miller, P. 'Empathy, sympathy and altruism: Empirical and conceptual', in *Empathy and Its Development* (eds) N. Eisenberg & J. Strayer (Cambridge: Cambridge University Press, 1987), pp. 292–316.

Eth, S. & Wesley Robb, J. 'Informed consent: The problem', in *Ethics in Mental Health Practice* (eds) Kentsmith, Miya & Salladay (Florida: Grune & Stratton, 1986), pp. 83–109.

Frankena, W. *Ethics* (NJ. USA : Prentice Hall, 1973).

Frey, R. G. 'Act-utilitarianism' in *Ethical Theory* (ed.) H. LaFollette (Oxford: Blackwell Publishers, 2000).

Fried, C. *Right and Wrong* (Cambridge, MA: Harvard University Press, 1978).

Garrard, E. 'Slote on virtue', *Analysis*, 2000, **60** (3), pp. 280–284.

Gauthier, D. *Morals by Agreement* (Oxford: Oxford University Press, 1986).

Geach, P. T. *The Virtues* (Cambridge: Cambridge University Press, 1977).

Gert, B. Culver, C. M. & Clouser, K. D. *Bioethics – a Return to Fundamentals* (New York: Oxford University Press, 1997).

Gibson, C. 'Ethical dilemmas faced by mental health nurses', *Nursing Standard* 1997, **11** (48), pp. 38–40.

Gillon, R. *Philosophical Medical Ethics* (Chichester: John Wiley & Sons, 1986).

Glaser, B. G. & Strauss, A. L. *The Discovery of Grounded Theory. Strategies for Qualitative Research* (Chicago: Aldine Press, 1967).

Glover, J. *Causing Death and Saving Lives* (Harmondsworth: Penguin, 1977).

Gregory, R. J. 'Recovery from depression associated with Guillain Barre Syndrome', *Issues in Mental Health Nursing*, 2003, **24** (2), pp. 129–135.

Griffin, J. *Wellbeing* (Oxford: Clarendon Press, 1986).

Haack, S. 'Pragmatism', in *A Companion to Epistemology* (eds) J. Dancy & E. Sosa (Oxford: Blackwells, 1992), pp. 351–357.

Hare, R. M. *Moral Thinking* (Oxford: Oxford University Press, 1981).

Healy, M. & Iles, J. 'The establishment and enforcement of codes', *Journal of Business Ethics*, 2002, **39** (1), pp. 117–124.

Hewitt, J. 'A critical review of the arguments debating the role of the nurse advocate', *Journal of Advanced Nursing*, 2002, **37** (5), pp. 439–445.

Hobbes, T. *Leviathan* (ed.) C. B. MacPherson (Harmondsworth: Penguin, 1985).

Hopkinson, J. B. Hallet, C. E. & Luker, K. A. 'Caring for dying people in hospital', *Journal of Advanced Nursing*, 2003, **44** (5), pp. 525–532.

Hopton, J. 'Control and restraint in contemporary psychiatric nursing: Some ethical considerations', *Journal of Advanced Nursing* 1995, **22,** pp. 110–115.

Horton, J. & Mendus, S. 'Alasdair MacIntyre: After Virtue and After', in *After MacIntyre – Critical Perspectives on the Work of Alasdair MacIntyre* (eds) Horton and Mendus (Cambridge: Polity Press, 1994).

Hume, D. *An Enquiry Concerning the Principles of Morals*, 3rd edn (ed.) L. A. Bigge & rev. P. H. Nidditch (Oxford: Clarendon Press, 1975).

Hunter, M. 'Rehabilitation in cancer care: A patient-focused approach', *European Journal of Cancer Care*, 1998, **7** (2), pp. 85–87;

Hurst, K. & Howard, D. 'Measure for measure', *Nursing Times*, 1988, **84** (22), pp. 30–32.

Hursthouse, R. 'Virtue theory and abortion', in *Virtue Ethics* (eds) R Crisp and M. Slote (Oxford: Oxford University Press, 1997), pp. 217–238.

Hursthouse, R. *On Virtue Ethics* (Oxford: Oxford University Press, 1999).

Ironbar, O. & Hooper, A. *Self Instruction in Mental Health Nursing*, 2nd edn (London: Balliere Tindall, 1989).

Irwin, T. *Greek Ethics* (Oxford: Oxford University Press, 1999).

Jackson, S. & Stevenson, C. 'The gift of time from the friendly professional', *Nursing Standard*, 1998, **12** (51), pp. 31–33.

Jaeger, S. Z. 'Teaching health care ethics: The importance of moral sensitivity for moral reasoning', *Nursing Philosophy*, 2001, **2**, pp. 131–143.

Johns, J. L. 'A concept analysis of trust', *Journal of Advanced Nursing*, 1996, **24**, pp. 76–83.

Johnson, L. *Focusing on Truth* (London: Routledge, 1992).

Johnstone, M. J. & Fry, S. T. *Ethics in Nursing Practice: A Guide to Ethical Decision-Making* (Oxford: Blackwells, 2002).

Jones, P. *Rights* (London: Macmillan, 1994).

Kadner, K. 'Therapeutic intimacy in nursing', *Journal of Advanced Nursing*, 1994, **19**, pp. 215–218.

Kant, I. 'Grounding for the Metaphysics of Morals', 2nd sec.: 429 trans. J. W. Ellington (Indianapolis: Hackett Publishing Company, 1981).

Kant, I. 'The doctrine of right', in *The Metaphysics of Morals* (ed.) M. Gregor (Cambridge: Cambridge University Press, 1996).

Kant, I. 'The doctrine of virtue', in *The Metaphysics of Morals* (ed.) M. Gregor (Cambridge: Cambridge University Press, 1996).

Kashka, M. S. & Keyser, P. K. 'Ethical issues in informed consent and ECT', *Perspectives in Psychiatric Care*, 1995, **31**, pp. 15–21.

Kenny, A. *Action, Emotion and Will* (London: Routledge, 1963).

Kentsmith, D. K., Miya, P. A. & Salladay, S. A. 'Decision-making in mental health practice', in *Ethics in Mental Health Practice* (eds) Kentsmith, Miya & Salladay (Florida: Grune & Stratton, 1986).

Kinion, E., S. Jonke, N. L. & Paradise, N. 'Descriptive ethics and neuroleptic drug reduction', *Perspectives in Psychiatric Care*, 1995, **31** (2), pp. 11–14.

Lacey, D. 'Using Orem's model in psychiatric nursing', *Nursing Standard*, 1993, **7** (29), pp. 28–30.

Latvala, E., Janhonen, S. & Wahlberg, K. E. 'Patient initiatives during the assessment and planning of psychiatric nursing in a hospital environment', *Journal of Advanced Nursing*, 1999, **29** (1), pp. 64–71.

Lessnoff, M. *Social Contract* (Oxford: Polity Press, 1988).

Llamas, K. J., Pickhauer, A. M. & Pillar, N. B. 'Mainstreaming palliative care for cancer patients in the acute hospital setting',*Palliative Medicine*, 2001, **15**, pp. 207–212.

Loubardias, S. 'Ethics of electroconvulsive therapy consent', *Rehabilitation Nursing*, 1991, **16** (2), pp. 98–100.

Louden, R. B. 'On some vices of virtue ethics', in *Virtue Ethics* (eds) R. Crisp & M. Slote (Oxford: Oxford University Press, 1997), pp. 201–216.

Lutzen, K. & Nordin, C. 'Benevolence, a central moral concept derived from a grounded theory study of nursing decision making in psychiatric settings', *Journal of Advanced Nursing*, 1993, **18**, pp. 1106–1111.

Lutzen, K., & Nordin, C. 'Structuring moral meaning in psychiatric nursing', *Scandinavian Journal of Caring Sciences*, 1993, **7**, pp. 175–180.

Lutzen, K. & Nordin, C. 'Modifying autonomy – a concept grounded in nurses' experiences of moral decision making in psychiatric practice', *Journal of Medical Ethics*, 1994, **20**, pp. 101–107.

Lutzen, K. & Barbosa da Silva, A. 'The role of virtue ethics in psychiatric nursing', *Nursing Ethics*, 1996, **3** (3) pp. 202–211.

Lyons, D. *Forms and Limits of Utilitarianism* (Oxford: Clarendon Press, 1965).

MacIntyre, A. *A Short History of Ethics* (London: Routledge and Kegan Paul, 1967).

MacIntyre, A. *Against the Self-Images of the Age: Essays on Ideology and Philosophy* (London: Duckworth, 1971).

MacIntyre, A. *After Virtue – A Study in Moral Theory*, 2nd edn (London: Duckworth, 1985).

MacIntyre, A. *Whose Justice? Which Rationality?* (London: Duckworth, 1988).

MacIntyre, A. 'A partial response to my critics', isn *After MacIntyre* (eds) J. Horton & S. Mendus (Cambridge: Polity Press, 1994).

MacIntyre, A. *Dependent Rational Animals – Why Humans Need the Virtues* (London: Duckworth, 1999).

Malaviya, A. N. 'Outcome measures in rheumatoid arthritis', *Journal of Rheumatology*, 2003, **6** (2), pp. 178–183.

Mallick, M. 'Advocacy in nursing – a review of the literature', *Journal of Advanced Nursing*, 1997, **25** (1), pp. 130–138.

Marck, P. 'Therapeutic reciprocity: A caring phenomenon', *Advances in Nursing Science*, 1990, **13**, pp. 49–59.

Marcus, B. 'Dilemma', in *The Oxford Companion to Philosophy* (ed.) T. Honderich (Oxford: Oxford University Press, 1995), p. 201.

Martin, G. W. 'Ritual action and its effect on the role of the nurse as advocate', *Journal of Advanced Nursing*, 1998, **27** (1), pp. 189–194.

Martin, T. 'Psychiatric nurses' use of working time', *Nursing Standard*, 1992, **6**, pp. 34–36.

Mason, A. 'MacIntyre on modernity and how it has marginalized the virtues', in *How Should One Live?* (ed.) R. Crisp (Oxford: Oxford University Press, 1996).

May, C. 'Research on nurse-patient relationships: Problems of theory, problems of practice', *Journal of Advanced Nursing* 1990, **15**, pp. 307–315.

McAlpine, H., Kristjanson, L. & Poroch, D. 'Development and testing of the ethical reasoning tool (ERT): An instrument to measure the ethical reasoning of nurses', *Journal of Advanced Nursing*, 1997, **25**, pp. 1151–1161.

McKie, A. & Swinton, J. 'Community, culture and character: The place of the virtues in psychiatric nursing practice', *Journal of Psychiatric and Mental Health Nursing*, 2000, **7**, pp. 35–42.

Menzies, I. 'A case study in the functioning of social systems as a defense against anxiety. A report on a study of the nursing service of a general hospital', *Human Relations*, 1960, **13** (2), pp. 95–121.

Mill, J. S. 'Utilitarianism', in *Classics of Western Philosophy* (ed.) S. M. Cahn (Indianapolis: Hackett Publishing Group, Inc. 1990), pp.1063–1114.

Mill, J. S. 'Utilitarianism', in *Utilitarianism* (ed.) R. Crisp (Oxford: Oxford University Press, 1998).

Miller, D. 'Virtues, practices and justice', in *After MacIntyre* (eds) J. Horton & S. Mendus (Cambridge: Polity Press, 1994).

Ming Ho Lau, V., & Mackenzie, A. 'Attributes of nurses that determine the quality of care for mentally handicapped people in an institution', *Journal of Advanced Nursing*, 1996, **24** (6), pp. 1109–1115.

Moir, J. & Abraham, C. 'Why I want to be a psychiatric nurse: Constructing an identity through contrasts with general nursing', *Journal of Advanced Nursing*, 1996, **23** (2), pp. 295–298.

Monaghan, A. 'Communication', in *Potter and Perry's Foundations in Nursing Theory and Practice* (ed.) H. B. M. Heath (London: Mosby, 1995), pp. 275–297.

Mulhall, S. & Swift, A. *Liberals and Communitarians* (Oxford: Blackwells, 1992).

Murdoch, I. *Sovereignty of Good* (London: Routledge & Kegan Paul, 1970).

Murphy, J. G. 'Repentance and Criminal Punishment', in *Ethics in Practice* (ed.) H. LaFollette (Cambridge, MA: Blackwells, 1997) pp. 487–493.

Murphy, K., Cooney, A., Casey, D., Connor, M., O'Connor, J. & Dineen, B. 'The Roper, Logan and Tierney model: Perceptions and operationalization of the model in psychiatric nursing within a health board in Ireland', *Journal of Advanced Nursing*, 2000, **31** (6), pp. 1333–1341.

Musker, M. & Byrne, M. 'Applying empowerment in mental health practice', *Nursing Standard*, 1997, **11** (31), pp. 45–47.

Nagel, T. *The View from Nowhere* (New York: Oxford University Press, 1986).

Nietzsche, F. *Beyond Good and Evil*, trans. Walter Kaufmann (New York: Vintage Books, 1966).

Nightingale, F. *Notes on Nursing: What It Is and What It Is Not* (New York: Dover Publications, 1969).

Norman, R. *The Moral Philosophers* (Oxford: Clarendon Press, 1983), pp. 37–55.

Nortvedt, P. 'Sensitive judgment: An inquiry into the foundations of nursing ethics', *Nursing Ethics*, 1998, **5** (5), pp. 385–392.

Nouwen, H. J., McNeill, D. P. & Morrison, D. A. *Compassion: A Reflection on the Christian Life* (London: Darton, Longman and Todd, 1982).

Nursing & Midwifery Council, *The Code of Professional Conduct: Standards for Conduct, Performance and Ethics* (London: NMC, 2004).

Nursing and Midwifery Council, *What Accountability Is* (London: NMC, 2002).

Nussbaum, M. C. 'Non-relative virtues: An Aristotelian approach', in *Midwest Studies in Philosophy, vol. XII: Ethical Theory: Character and Virtue* (eds) P. A. French, T. E. Vehling Jr. & H. K. Wettstein (Notre Dame: University of Notre Dame Press, 1988), pp. 32–53.

Nussbaum, M. 'Compassion: The basic social emotion', *Social Philosophy and Policy Foundation*, 1996, **13**, pp. 27–58.

Oakley, J. *Morality and the Emotions* (London: Routledge, 1992).

Oakley, J. & Cocking, D. *Virtue Ethics and Professional Roles* (Cambridge: Cambridge University Press, 2001).

O'Neill, O. *Abstraction, Idealization and Ideology in Ethics* (Cambridge: Cambridge University Press, 1987).

O'Neill, O. 'Kant's ethics', in *A Companion to Ethics* (ed.) P. Singer (Oxford: Blackwells, 1991), pp. 175–185.

Orlando, I. *The Dynamic Nurse–Patient Relationship* (New York: Putnam & Sons, 1961).

Parsons, S., Barker, P. J. & Armstrong, A. E. 'The teaching of health care ethics to students of nursing in the UK: A pilot study', *Nursing Ethics*, 2001, **8** (1), pp. 45–56.

Pearson, A. 'Trends in clinical nursing', in *Primary Nursing. Nursing in the Burford and Oxford Nursing Development Units* (ed.) A. Pearson (London: Croon Helm, 1988), pp.1–122.

Pellegrino, E. & Thomasma, D. C. *A Philosophical Basis of Medical Practice* (New York: Oxford University Press, 1981).

Pellegrino, E. & Thomasma, D. C. *For the Patient's Good* (New York: Oxford University Press, 1988).

Pellegrino, E. & Thomasma, D. C. *The Virtues in Medical Practice* (New York: Oxford University Press, 1993).

Pence, G. 'Virtue theory', in *A Companion to Ethics* (ed.) P. Singer (Oxford: Blackwells, 1991), p. 249–259.

Penn, K. 'Patient advocacy in palliative care', *British Journal of Nursing*, 1994, **3**, 1, pp. 40–42.

Peplau, H. *Interpersonal Relations in Nursing* (New York: Putnam, 1952).

Peter, E. & Morgan, K. P. 'Explorations of a trust approach for nursing ethics', *Nursing Inquiry*, 2001, **8**, pp. 3–10.

Pettit, P. 'The consequentialist perspective', in *Three Methods of Ethics* (Oxford: Blackwells, 1997), pp. 92–174.

Pincoffs, E. *Quandaries and Virtues: Against Reductivism in Ethics* (Lawrence: University of Kansas Press, 1986).

Pincoffs, E. 'Quandary ethics', in *Ethical Theory 2 – Theories about How We Should Live* (ed.) J. Rachels (New York: Oxford University Press, 1998), pp.187–205.

Plato, *Meno*, in *Protagoras and Meno* trans. W. K. C. Guthrie (London: Penguin Books, 1956).

Rachels, J. 'Punishment and desert', in *Ethics in Practice* (ed.) H. LaFollette (Cambridge, MA: Blackwells, 1997), pp. 470–479.

Rachels, J. *The Elements of Moral Philosophy*, 3rd edn (New York: McGraw-Hill, 1999).

Ramos, M. C. 'The nurse–patient relationship: Theme and variation', *Journal of Advanced Nursing*, 1992, **17**, pp. 496–506.

Ramussen, D. B. 'Human flourishing and the appeal to human nature', in *Human Flourishing* (eds) E. F. Paul, F. D. Miller Jr & J. Paul (New York: Cambridge University Press, 1999), pp. 1–43.

Randers, I. & Mattrasson, A. C. 'Autonomy and integrity: Upholding older adult patients' dignity', *Journal of Advanced Nursing*, 2004, **45** (1), pp. 63–71.

Raphael, D. D. *Moral Philosophy* 2nd edn (Oxford: Oxford University Press, 1994).

Rawls, J. *A Theory of Justice* (Cambridge, MA: Harvard University Press, 1971).

Rescher, N. *The Coherence Theory of Truth* (Oxford: Oxford University Press, 1973).

Rescher, N. *Rationality: A Philosophical Inquiry into the Nature and the Rationale of Reason* (Oxford: Oxford University Press, 1988).

Rest, J. 'A psychologist looks at the teaching of ethics', *The Hastings Centre Report*, 1982, **12**, pp. 29–36.

Rorty, R. *The Consequences of Pragmatism* (Hassocks: Harvester, 1982).

Ross, W. D. *The Right and the Good* (Oxford: Clarendon Press, 1930).

'Rule utilitarianism', in *The Internet Encyclopaedia of Philosophy* (author unknown), www.utm.edu/research/iep/r/ruleutil.htm, last accessed 12/1/02.

Sanson–Fischer, R., Poole, A. & Thompson, V. 'Behaviour patterns within a general hospital psychiatric unit: An observational study', *Behaviour Research and Therapy*, 1979, **17**, pp. 317–332.

Salladay, S. A. 'Ethical responsibility in mental health practice', in *Ethics in Mental Health Practice* (eds) Kentsmith, Miya & Salladay (Florida: Grune & Stratton, 1986).

Scheffler, S. *Human Morality* (Oxford: Oxford University Press, 1992.)

Scott, P. A. 'Emotion, moral perception and nursing practice', *Nursing Philosophy* 2000, **1**, pp. 123–133.

Sellman, D. 'Alasdair MacIntyre and the professional practice of nursing', *Nursing Philosophy*, 2000, **1**, pp. 26–33.

Sidgwick, H. *The Methods of Ethics* (London: Macmillan, 1962).

Skidmore, D. 'Communication', in *A Textbook of Psychiatric and Mental Health Nursing* (eds) J. I. Brooking, S. A. H. Ritter & B. L. Thomas (Edinburgh: Churchill Livingstone, 1992), pp. 249–259.

Skinner, B. F. *Science and Human Behaviour* (New York: Macmillan, 1953).

Slote, M. *From Morality to Virtue* (New York: Oxford University Press, 1992).

Slote, M. 'Agent-based virtue ethics', in *Virtue Ethics* (eds) R. Crisp & M. Slote (Oxford: Oxford University Press, 1997), pp. 239–262.

Slote, M. *Morals with Motives* (Oxford: Oxford University Press, 2001).

Smart, J. J. C. 'An outline of a system of utilitarian ethics', in *Utilitarianism For and Against* (Cambridge: Cambridge University Press, 1973), pp. 3–67.

Snelson, C. 'Trust as a caring construct with the critically ill: A beginning exploration', in *The Presence of Caring in Nursing* (ed.) D. A. Gaut (New York: National League for Nursing Press, 1992).

Speedy, S. 'The therapeutic alliance', in *Advanced Practice in Mental Health Nursing* (eds) M. Clinton & S. Nelson (Oxford: Blackwell Science, 1999), pp. 59–76.

Stocker, M. 'The schizophrenia of modern ethical theories', in *Virtue Ethics* (eds) R. Crisp & M. Slote (Oxford: Oxford University Press, 1997), pp. 66–78.

232   *Bibliography*

Stohr, K. & Wellman, C. H. 'Recent work on virtue ethics', *American Philosophical Quarterly,* 2002, **39** (1), pp. 49–71.

Strang, J. *The Emotional Labour of Nursing* (London: Macmillan Press, 1982).

Sumner, L. *The Moral Foundation of Rights* (Oxford: Clarendon Press, 1987).

Swanton, C. 'Virtue ethics and satisficing rationality', in *Virtue Ethics – A Critical Reader* (ed.) D. Statman (Edinburgh: Edinburgh University Press, 1997), pp. 56–81.

Tarbuck, P. 'Ethical standards and human rights', *Nursing Standard* 1992, **7** (6), 27–30.

Tarbuck, P. 'Use and abuse of control and restraint', *Nursing Standard,* 1992, **6** (52), pp. 30–32.

Thompson, D. (ed.) 'Knowledge', in *Oxford Compact English Dictionary* (Oxford: Oxford University Press, 1996), p. 549.

Tilley, S. 'Notes on narrative knowledge in psychiatric nursing', *Journal of Psychiatric & Mental Health Nursing,* 1995, **2** (4), pp. 217–226.

Travelbee, J. *Interpersonal Aspects of Nursing,* (Philadelphia: F. A. Davis, 1966).

Tsay, S. L. & Hung, L. O. 'Empowerment of patients with end stage renal disease – a randomized controlled trial', *International Journal of Nursing Studies,* 2004, **41** (1), pp. 59–65.

Tschudin, V. *Ethics in Nursing – the Caring Relationship,* 3rd edn (Oxford: Butterworth Heinmann, 2003).

Tuckett, A. G. 'An ethic of the fitting: A conceptual framework for nursing practice', *Nursing Inquiry,* 1998, **5**, pp. 220–227.

von Dietze, E. & Orb, A. 'Compassionate care: A moral dimension of nursing', *Nursing Inquiry,* 2000, **7**, pp. 166–174.

Walker, L., Barker, P. J. & Pearson, P. 'The required role of the psychiatric-mental health nurse in primary health care: An augmented Delphi study', *Nursing Inquiry,* 2000, **7**, pp. 91–102.

Walsh, M. & Ford, P. *Nursing Rituals, Research and Rational Actions* (Oxford: Butterworth Heinemann, 1994).

Ward, M. 'The consequences of service planning in mental health nursing', in *Ethical Issues in Mental Health* (eds) P. J. Barker & S. Baldwin (Cheltenham: Stanley Thornes, 1997), pp. 127–147.

Whittington, D. & McLaughlin, C. 'Finding time for patients: An exploration of nurses' time allocation in an acute psychiatric setting', *Journal of Psychiatric and Mental Health Nursing,* 2000, **7**, pp. 259–268.

Williams, B. *Moral Luck* (Cambridge: Cambridge University Press, 1981).

Williams, B. *Ethics and the Limits of Philosophy* (London: Fontana Press, 1985).

Williams, B. *Making Sense of Humanity* (Cambridge: Cambridge University Press, 1995).

Woods, S. 'Holism in nursing', in *Philosophical Issues in Nursing* (ed.) S. D. Edwards (London: Macmillan, 1998), pp. 67–88.

Wright, H. 'The therapeutic relationship', in *Mental Health Nursing* (eds) H. Wright & M. Giddey (London: Chapman & Hall, 1993), pp. 3–9.

Yegdich, T. 'On the phenomenology of empathy in nursing: Empathy or sympathy?', *Journal of Advanced Nursing* 1999, **30** (1), pp. 83–93.

Zakrzewski, R. F. & Hector, M. A. 'The lived experiences of alcohol addiction: Men of Alcoholics Anonymous', *Issues in Mental Health Nursing,* 2004, **25** (1), pp. 61–77.

Index

240   *Index*

practice – *continued*
patients who have committed
deplorable acts 150–2
reasons for action 147–8
virtues 26–39
action-guidance 37–8
conflicts between 102–5, 153–5, 194
definitions 30, 34–5
excessive 152–3
'goodness' 30–1
identification of 31–2, 38–9
MacIntyre 157–79
obligations-based approach 122–3
principlism 120
research findings 15–16

role of the nurse 19
universality 33–4
value of 35–6
vulnerability 7–9, 11, 24, 137, 146

Webster, C. 9
welfarist theory 42, 43
well-being 42–3, 70, 72, 84
Whitehill, I. 20
Whittington, D. 22
Williams, B. 45
'wrong'
consequentialism 41, 59
deontology 60, 67–8
virtue ethics 82, 99
virtues 37

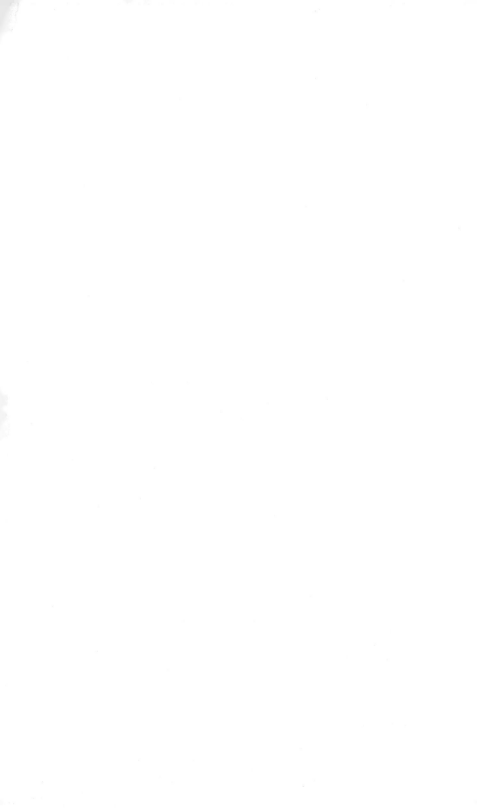

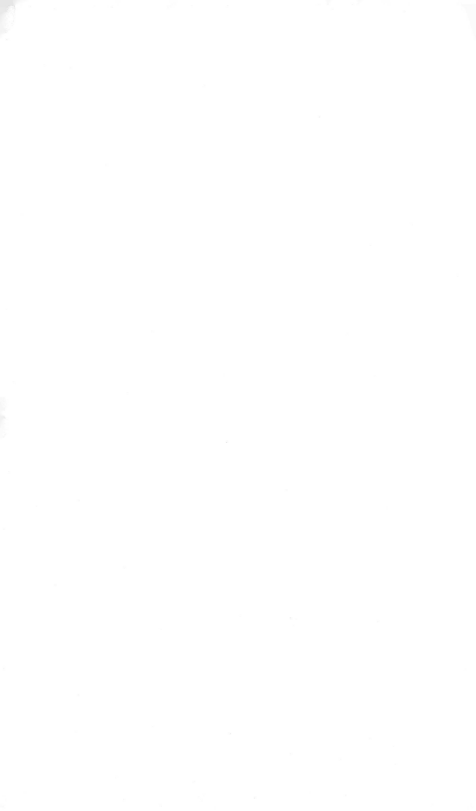